PRACTICING RIGHTS

Professional social work Codes of Ethics around the world appeal to the concept of people having "rights" that social workers need to respect and advocate for. However, it isn't always clear how social workers can actually incorporate human rights-based approaches in their practice, whether domestic or international. This book fills this gap by advancing rights-based approaches to social work.

The first part gives an overview of the relationship between human rights and social work, and outlines a model for how rights-based approaches can be integrated into social work practice. The second part introduces the rights-based framework across five mainstream areas of practice – poverty, child welfare, older adults, health, and mental health. Each of these substantive chapters:

- introduces the area of practice and traditional social welfare interventions associated with it
- outlines relevant human rights frameworks
- explores case studies showcasing rights-based approaches
- presents practical implications for implementing rights-based social work practice.

The book ends with a discussion of the limitations and criticisms of rights-based approaches and lays out some future directions for practice.

This accessible text is designed for all those interested in learning how to introduce human rights-based interventions into their practice. It will be of particular use to social work students taking direct practice, macro practice, social policy, international social work, and human rights courses as part of their program.

David Androff, MSW, Ph.D., is an Associate Professor in the School of Social Work at Arizona State University where he is Associate Director of the Office of Global Social Work and a Senior Sustainability Scholar with the Julie Ann Wrigley Global Institute of Sustainability. He earned his Masters and Ph.D. in Social Welfare from the University of California, Berkeley. Dr. Androff's interests center on building strong and sustainable communities through promoting human rights. His scholarship explores the connections between human rights and social work and has investigated Truth and Reconciliation Commissions, refugee empowerment, immigration policy, and human trafficking. Dr. Androff's scholarship was recognized with the 2011 Emerging Scholar Award from the Association of Community Organization and Social Administration. He is a founding member of the CSWE Committee on Human Rights.

PRACTICING RIGHTS

Human rights-based approaches to social work practice

David Androff

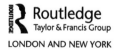

Routledge
Taylor & Francis Group

LONDON AND NEW YORK

First published 2016
by Routledge
2 Park Square, Milton Park, Abingdon, Oxon OX14 4RN

and by Routledge
711 Third Avenue, New York, NY 10017

Routledge is an imprint of the Taylor & Francis Group, an informa business

© 2016 D. Androff

British Library Cataloguing in Publication Data
A catalogue record for this book is available from the British Library

Library of Congress Cataloging-in-Publication Data
Androff, David K., author.
   Practicing rights : human rights-based approaches to social work practice / written by David K. Androff.
      pages cm
   Includes bibliographical references and index.
   1. Social service—Practice.   2. Social workers—Professional ethics.   3. Social service—Moral and ethical aspects.   4. Human rights.   I. Title.
   [DNLM: 1. Social Work.   2. Human Rights.   3. Internationality. 4. Vulnerable Populations.   HV 40]
   HV10.5.A523 2016
   361.3'2—dc23
   2015005342

ISBN: 978-0-415-70953-8 (hbk)
ISBN: 978-0-415-70954-5 (pbk)
ISBN: 978-1-315-88548-3 (ebk)

Typeset in Bembo
by Apex CoVantage, LLC

This book is dedicated to my mother
Margaret Aletha Wilkerson Androff

CONTENTS

PREFACE

After delivering a presentation on human rights at the Asian and Pacific Association of Social Work Education conference in Manila, a young Filipino social worker in the audience raised her hand and said, "Thank you for this excellent information, but can you give us a specific example of how we can apply human rights to our practice?" My answer became this book.

Human rights have been identified as fundamental to social work. Indeed the profession shares many of its priorities, ethical values, and even historical development with the field of human rights. Despite this, there has been relatively little attention given to the relationship of human rights to professional practice in social work. At the same time, human rights-based approaches have been growing in popularity for addressing pressing social problems around the globe. Non-governmental organizations in the fields of international development and public health are increasingly modifying their work based on the principles of human rights. The United Nations (UN) has begun to mainstream human rights into all of its work, while UN agencies such as the UNDP and UNICEF have already implemented rights-based approaches. However, social work and the related helping professions have yet to identify rights-based approaches to practice.

Attention to human rights issues in the social work literature is growing. Social work literature on human rights introduces practitioners to human rights, emphasizes the importance of human rights theory and documents for practitioners, draws attention to human rights issues, and encourages professionals to make use of human rights. While this literature notes the potential for human rights to influence social work, it does not present approaches to practice. To date there has been no exploration or presentation of a human rights approach to social work practice. In this way, the link between human rights and social work remains underdeveloped.

This book addresses this gap by advancing the literature on human rights through an examination of their potential for professional social work practice in core social work domains. The book begins with two chapters that set the context for rights-based approaches to social work practice. The first chapter assesses the current status of human rights within social work and argues for the relevance of human rights to professional practice. The second chapter presents a theoretical framework for human rights-based practice that is drawn from human rights principles of human dignity, nondiscrimination, participation, transparency, and accountability.

The heart of the book is the middle five chapters that carry the framework of human rights principles for practice across several key domains of professional practice, including poverty, child welfare, older adults, health, and mental health. These chapters are structured similarly, including overviews of the field and traditional approaches for context, pertinent human rights standards, case studies that illuminate rights-based approaches in practice, and implications for rights-based social work practice. These chapters focus on a distinct practice area or population; practice domains have been selected specifically to strengthen the argument that rights-based approaches are applicable to traditional social work practice settings. Hot-button human rights topics such as trafficking have been purposefully avoided. These particular five areas also represent core human rights fields, across the three generations of rights.

Poverty was chosen as one of the chief problems that social work professionals confront in many dimensions of practice; also rights-based approaches to poverty in the field of international development have become established and it is therefore a natural choice to begin linking rights-based approaches with social work. In order to demonstrate the utility of rights-based approaches across the life span and to two populations of central concern to social workers, the next two chapters focus on child welfare and older adults. The two chapters that follow focus on health and mental health, which should also appeal to mainstream social work practitioners and policymakers. The chapter on health incorporates innovations from global public health and the chapter on mental health includes important contributions from the disability rights field as well as the recovery movement.

The final chapter discusses the perils and prospects of applying rights-based approaches to social work. These concluding reflections acknowledge the limitations of adopting rights-based approaches to social work practice by addressing critiques of human rights, and point to future directions for human rights in social work.

ACKNOWLEDGMENTS

It is my deep pleasure to acknowledge my debts to several people; this book would not have been possible without the support of many. I am truly standing on the shoulders of giants. I am primarily indebted to James Midgley, my doctoral mentor who continues to support and inspire me. Professor Midgley nurtured my unorthodox research pursuits, and taught me, by example and direction, to pursue big ideas in my scholarship. My social work education at the University of California, Berkeley was enriched by my studies at the Human Rights Center, in particular with Professors Harvey Weinstein and Vincent Iacopino.

My perspective on social work and human rights was shaped by my experiences as a social worker practicing in human rights settings. I am grateful for the support of the California Office of the State Public Defender and for teaching me how much a social worker can contribute to human rights. I am indebted to the Timor-Leste Commission for Reception, Truth, and Reconciliation and the Timorese people for teaching me about human rights and their limits "on the ground".

I have been fortunate to have had the opportunity to collaborate with amazing colleagues. It is indeed an exciting time to be working in the area of human rights and social work. I have benefited tremendously from the community of scholars laboring to advance human rights in social work. I am particularly grateful to Kathy Libal, Scott Harding, Shirley Gatenio Gabel, Meghan Berthold, and Susan Mapp for their encouragement and support. Special mention goes to my friend and collaborator Jane McPherson, to whom I am grateful for her enthusiasm and energy. At Arizona State University, I have been grateful for the support and camaraderie of the Southwest Collaborative on Immigration, Inequality, and Poverty which has spurred my scholarship on human rights and immigration.

I am indebted to Grace McInnes at Routledge for her vision, persistence, and faith in this project. James Watson and Louisa Vahtrick have also assisted me along my way.

Most of all, I am grateful for the love of my wife Jill Messing, whose boundless support has contributed immeasurably to my life and to this book. Our daughters provide me with unending light and truth, and prevent me from taking myself too seriously. I am especially grateful to my parents for their constant love and support.

ABOUT THE AUTHOR

David Androff, MSW, Ph.D., is an Associate Professor in the School of Social Work at Arizona State University where he is Associate Director of the Office of Global Social Work and a Senior Sustainability Scholar with the Julie Ann Wrigley Global Institute of Sustainability. He earned his Masters and Ph.D. in Social Welfare from the University of California, Berkeley. Dr. Androff's interests center on building strong and sustainable communities through promoting human rights. His scholarship explores the connections between human rights and social work and has investigated Truth and Reconciliation Commissions, refugee empowerment, immigration policy, and human trafficking. Dr. Androff's scholarship was recognized with the 2011 Emerging Scholar Award from the Association of Community Organization and Social Administration. He is a founding member of the CSWE Committee on Human Rights.

1

THE RELEVANCE OF HUMAN RIGHTS TO SOCIAL WORK

Human rights are a critically important means to protecting people from abuse and oppression. Many people engaged in human rights work are on the front lines of protecting vulnerable populations. This is true of social workers, who labor to improve the quality of life of people, to prevent, minimize, or ameliorate social problems, and to maximize human potential. Social workers are said to be doing human rights work, insofar as they are responsible for implementing political, civil, economic, social, and cultural rights, and increasingly environmental rights. Yet the two fields lack awareness of each other; both sets of professionals ignore each other's practice tools even as they grasp towards each other. The social work profession has embraced the rhetoric of human rights and has much in common with human rights, yet there remains significant divergence between the two fields. How can the social work profession avail itself of human rights to strengthen social work practice?

This chapter makes the case for the relevance of human rights to social work. The main focus of this chapter is upon analyzing social work's relationship to human rights, and exploring the basis of social work as a human rights profession. The first section concerns the current emphasis upon human rights within the social work profession. This includes a review of the ethical codes and statements of major professional organizations that reference human rights, the recent major scholarly and educational publications with a focus on human rights, the major professional conferences and meetings with a focus on human rights, curricula developments relating to human rights, and the *Global Agenda for Social Work and Social Development*'s relationship to human rights. It presents overlapping histories and priorities between the two fields and examines the gaps that separate them. The chapter demonstrates that human rights are an idea whose time has come in social work and examines the ways in which human rights and social work converge. Excavation of the common ground between human rights and social work builds the case that these fields could be and should be better integrated, therefore raising the importance of identifying and incorporating rights-based approaches to social work practice.

The relevance of human rights to social work is that it can make social work more relevant. This book aims to promote rights-based approaches to social work practice. This chapter contains the rationale for this book by outlining the potential for rights-based practice approaches to revitalize social work and to bring the profession to greater prominence in society and closer to its own social justice commitments. This chapter ends with a brief discussion of the book's methodology.

The state of human rights in social work

There is growing attention to human rights from within social work. Several recent examples include the ethical statements of professional organizations, the global definition of social work, the development of the *Global Agenda for Social Work and Social Development*, international conference themes, curricula developments, and rapidly expanding publications including journal articles, books, edited volumes, and dissertations.

Definitions

In a 1988 Policy Statement on Human Rights, the International Federation of Social Workers (IFSW) proclaimed that "social work has, from its conception, been a human rights profession, having as its basic tenet the intrinsic value of every human being and as one of its main aims the promotion of equitable social structures, which can offer people security and development while upholding their dignity" (IFSW, 1988, introduction; UN, 1994, p. 3; Wronka, 2008). The 2000 international definition of social work adopted by the IFSW and the International Association of Schools of Social Work (IASSW) includes in its final line the statement that "principles of human rights and social justice are fundamental to social work" (IFSW & IASSW, 2000). This was the first time that human rights were explicitly linked to the definition of social work, and was influential. This definition became widely cited, and as the product of a process of compromise and consensus, this definition was criticized for including the human rights perspective as a bias towards Western and individualistic approaches, and another period of review, consultation, deliberation, and consensus was launched to revise the definition. In 2014 at the Joint World Conference of Social Work and Social Development in Melbourne, three of the major international social work professional organizations, the IASSW, IFSW, and the International Council of Social Welfare (ICSW) endorsed a new definition with the revised statement that "principles of social justice, human rights, collective responsibility, and respect for diversities are central to social work" (IASSW, IFSW & ICSW, 2014).

Global Agenda

In an effort to unify and amplify the voice of the global social work profession for greater impact and advocacy globally and locally, the IASSW, the IFSW and the

ICSW, in consultation with social workers around the world, developed the *Global Agenda for Social Work and Social Development* in 2012. The *Global Agenda* has as one of its four core themes "Promoting the dignity and worth of people", which is framed in terms of human rights. The *Global Agenda* calls for the "universal implementation of the international conventions and other instruments on social, economic, cultural and political rights for all peoples, including, among others, the rights of children, older people, women, persons with disabilities, and indigenous peoples, and the end to discrimination on the grounds of race and sexual orientation" (IASWW, IFSW & ICSW, 2012, p. 3).

Codes of Ethics

Human rights have been explicitly linked to social work in the Codes of Ethics of professional social work organizations that provide guidance for the field. Scholars have explored the ethical correlations between human rights and social work (Albrithen & Androff, 2015).

Globally

The International Federation of Social Workers' (IFSW) *Statement of Ethical Principles* (2012) notes the principles of human rights as central to social work, and conventions on human rights as relevant to social work. Human rights and human dignity are among the core ethical principles, meaning self-determination, participation, treating each person as a whole, and identifying and developing strengths.

North America

The Canadian Association of Social Workers' (CASW) *Code of Ethics* (2005) makes several explicit references to human rights in its ethical values of respect for the inherent dignity and worth of persons, including the directive to "uphold human rights" (CASW, 2005, p. 4). The U.S. professional organization, the National Association of Social Workers (NASW), does not mention human rights in its *Code of Ethics* (2008). However the term "rights" does appear in two places. It appears under social workers' ethical responsibilities to clients (1.14) which states that practitioners must "safeguard the interests and rights" of clients who "lack the capacity to make informed decisions". It also appears under social workers' ethical responsibilities to the broader society for social and political action (6.04), which includes among others the directive to "promote policies that safeguard the rights of and confirm equity and social justice for all people". This is not surprising given the cultural reluctance of the U.S. to embrace the language of human rights in the last few decades. However, the NASW *Code of Ethics* has been identified as aligning with the ideals and principles of human rights (Albrithen & Androff, 2015). Furthermore, NASW has endorsed "the fundamental principles set forth in the human rights documents of the United Nations" and encouraged the adoption of human rights as the "foundation principle upon which all social work theory and applied knowledge rests" (Falk, 1999, p. 17).

Pacific

The Australian Association of Social Workers (AASW) includes human rights in the definition of social work with the statement that "principles of human rights and social justice are fundamental to social work" (AASW, 2010, p. 7). It also includes among the commitments and aims of social work "working to achieve human rights and social justice through social development, social and systemic change, advocacy and the ethical conduct of research" by "subscribing to the principles and aspirations" of human rights (AASW, 2010, p. 7). Human rights is listed as a core social work value, linked to respect for persons and social justice (noted as both civil–political and economic–social–cultural). Among social workers' ethical responsibilities of respect for human dignity and worth is the directive that "social workers will respect others' beliefs, religious or spiritual world views, values, culture, goals, needs and desires, as well as kinship and communal bonds, within a framework of social justice and human rights". The AASW *Code of Ethics* lists the commitment to social justice and human rights as an ethical responsibility for all social workers; this responsibility is detailed to encompass participation, nondiscrimination, empowerment, transparency, self-determination, development, collective rights, and advocacy. In their responsibility to colleagues, social workers are mandated to acknowledge religious, spiritual, and secular diversity within a framework of social justice and human rights. The Aotearoa New Zealand Association of Social Workers' (ANZASW) *Code of Ethics* (2013) has a chapter on "Human Rights: International Conventions and Domestic Agencies" and mandates that practitioners protect clients' rights.

Europe

European social workers have long embraced human rights as a foundational aspect for practice. The European regional body of IFSW has a publication called *Standards in Social Work Practice meeting Human Rights* (2010) which extensively discusses how social workers should promote and realize human rights. It also sets out that "responding to human rights is the responsibility of the social work practitioner and social work educator". The British Association of Social Workers' (BASW) *Code of Ethics* (2012) lists respect for human rights as one of the core values and ethical principles for social workers practicing throughout the world, as the "motivation and justification for social work action" (BASW, 2012, p. 5). The *Code* refers to "the inherent worth and dignity of all people as expressed in the Universal Declaration of Human Rights (UN, 1948) and other related UN declarations on rights and the conventions derived from those declarations" (BASW, 2012, p. 8). The value of human rights is detailed to include the principles of human dignity and well-being, self-determination, participation, treating each person as a whole, and identifying and developing strengths. Social workers are mandated to use their authority "in accordance with human rights principles" (p. 13) and to "challenge the abuse of human rights" (p. 14). The Union of Social Educators and Social Workers of Russia (USESW) has an Ethical Guideline of Social Educator and Social Worker (USESW, 2003) that identifies human rights as related to the ethical values of human dignity and tolerance, social justice and humanism, the definition of social work, and the "motivation and legal ground of social work" (p. 19) in addition to including the Universal Declaration and subsequent human rights conventions on civil and political rights, racial discrimination, discrimination against women, and the rights of children.

Asia

The Japanese Association of Certified Social Workers (JACSW) has an ethical code (2004) that defines social work as related to human rights. It mandates social workers to collaborate in solidarity with international social workers and the international community to address international problems related to human rights and social justice. The *Code* further requires that social worker educators and researchers respect the human rights of students and practitioners as an ethical responsibility to society and a professional responsibility (JACSW, 2004). The Singapore Association of Social Workers' (SASW) *Code of Professional Ethics* mandates practitioners to respect and safeguard the rights of their clients (SASW, 1999). The Korean Association of Social Workers' (KASW) *Code of Ethics* lists "respect human rights and equality of every person" among the ethical standards with society for social workers (KASW, 2001, p. 5).

Latin America

The Asociación de Asistentes Sociales del Uruguay has a *Code of Ethics* (2014) that refers to human rights and the Universal Declaration of Human Rights.

Committees

The IFSW has had a standing Human Rights Commission since 1988 which advocates for the rights of social workers facing persecution; it has defended social workers against violence in East Timor, South Africa, Guatemala, Colombia, and the U.S. (Albrithen & Androff, 2015). In 2002 the IASSW and IFSW partnered to form a Joint Commission on Human Rights. In 2013 the Commission for Global Social Work Education (CSWE) formed a Committee on Human Rights.

Scholarship

The last decade has seen a rapid increase in scholarship on human rights and social work. This brief review of the most recent scholarship on human rights in the social work literature demonstrates the increased attention that human rights is receiving in many of the core social work practice and policy domains.

Books

Jim Ife's groundbreaking book on human rights and social work explored the philosophical and theoretical connections between the two fields and is now in its third edition (2012). Elisabeth Reichert's text introduced social workers to human rights standards and documents and is now in its second edition (2011). Reichert subsequently developed a classroom companion for students (2006) and an edited volume that explores several social work themes in human rights (2007). Joseph Wronka (2008) has detailed the historical development of human rights and social justice, linking both to social work practice. Susan Mapp's summary of global human rights issues for social workers is now in its second edition (2014). Colleen Lundy incorporated human rights into her work on structural social work practice, and this is in its second edition (2011). Shirley Gatenio Gabel is editing a series of texts on human rights and social work practice areas, including clinical practice (Berthold, 2015) and community practice (Libal & Harding, 2015). Several recent textbooks on international social work have included a heavy emphasis upon human rights and rights-related issues (Cox & Pawar, 2006; Healy, 2008a) as well as introduction to social work texts (van Wormer, 2006). Recent handbooks on international social work have also incorporated human rights chapters (Lyons, Hokenstad, Pawar, Huegler & Hall, 2012) and units on human rights (Healy & Link, 2012).

Articles in academic journals

In addition to books there has been a steady growth in peer-reviewed academic journal articles on human rights topics, or written from a human rights perspective, that make explicit reference to or use of human rights conventions, standards, or concepts. A search of the research database Social Service Abstracts for "human rights" and "social work" returned over 600 results. The rest of this section attempts to group the most explicit human rights-related articles in the social work literature since 2008.

The geographical range of these articles spans the globe, including Africa, Asia, and Latin America, as well as Europe and North America. This scholarship explores the relationship between social work and human rights (Ife, 2001; Solas, 2000; van Wormer, 2005; Witkin, 1998; Yu, 2006) as well as recovers their shared history (Healy, 2008b) and discusses the potential for integrating human rights with social work education and research (Chen, Tang & Lui, 2013; Dewees & Roche, 2001; George, 1999; Hawkins & Knox, 2014; McPherson & Abell, 2012; Steen, 2012; Steen & Mathiesen, 2005; Witkin, 1994). Much of the literature emphasizes macro practice, systems issues, policy, and advocacy (Cemlyn, 2008a; Ellis, 2004; Grodofsky, 2012; Holscher & Berhane, 2008; Ife & Fiske, 2006; Lombard, 2000; Lundy & van Wormer, 2007; Noyoo, 2004; Pyles, 2006; Steen, 2006; Watkinson, 2001). Other articles address core human rights debates, such as the tension between universalism and relativism, and the relationship between culture, human rights, and indigenization (Healy, 2007; Healy & Kamya, 2014; Katiuzhinsky & Okech, 2014; Sewpaul, 2007; Skegg, 2005; Staub-Bernasconi, 2011; Webb, 2009).

Most of this scholarship has focused on vulnerable populations central to social work, especially children (Ainsworth & Hansen, 2012; Ayinagadda, 2013; Hagues, 2013; Korr, Fallon & Brieland, 1994; Markward, 1999; Powell, Geoghegan, Scanlon & Swirak, 2013; Reynaert, Bouverne-De Bie & Vandevelde, 2010; Rotabi & Bromfield, 2012; Secker, 2013; Viviers & Lombard, 2013; Young, McKenzie, Schjelderup & Omre, 2012; Zavirsek & Herath, 2010) and also older adults (Patterson, 2004; Tang & Lee, 2006). Additional articles incorporate a gender perspective by addressing topics such as human rights and feminism (Dominelli, 1998; Reichert, 1998), poverty among women (Twill & Fisher, 2010), violence against women (Critelli, 2010; Morgaine, 2007), and reproductive rights (Alzate, 2009). Social work scholars have also used human rights to frame scholarship on other core domains of social work concern and social policy such as health (Fish & Bewley, 2010; Nadkarni, 2008; Ren, Washburn & Kao, 2013; Sulman, Kanee, Stewart & Savage, 2007; Williams, Vibbert, Mitchell & Serwanga, 2009), disability (Buchanan & Gunn, 2007; Fawcett & Plath, 2014; Kim, 2010; Leslie, 2008; Parker, 2006; Stainton, 2002), poverty (Jewell, Collins, Gargotto & Dishon, 2009; Townsend, 2006), criminal justice (Hounmenou, 2012; Mooradian, 2012), housing (van Wormer & van Wormer, 2009), and minority populations (Cemlyn, 2008b).

Scholarship has emerged applying human rights lenses to international social work topics and on social work practice with global populations such as on immigration (Androff, 2014; Androff & Tavassoli, 2012; Briskman & Cemlyn, 2005; Cemlyn & Briskman, 2003; Sanders et al., 2013; Zorn, 2009), refugees (Harding & Libal, 2012), and human trafficking (Androff, 2011; Bromfield & Rotabi, 2012). Another related focus is on international social work travel and exchanges (Ericson, 2011; Gammonley, Rotabi, Forte & Martin, 2013). Social work scholars have begun to address topics that have been traditionally thought of as primarily human rights topics, such as torture (Engstrom & Okamura, 2004), Truth and Reconciliation Commissions (Androff, 2010), religion (Hodge, 2006; Hodge, 2012), and environmental rights (Androff, Fike & Rorke, in press). Not all of the scholarship has been academic or aimed at students; Linda Briskman and colleagues published a *Report of the People's Inquiry Into Detention* (2006) that analyzed human rights violations among Australian immigration detention policies and facilities.

Conferences and meetings

Recent international and high profile social work conferences have featured human rights among its agenda topics and themes. The 2012 Joint World Conference on Social Work and Social Development in Stockholm had as one of its three core themes "Human rights and social equality" that posed the question "How can social work and social policies contribute in the endeavor to respect, protect, and fulfill human rights?" The 2013 18th Symposium of the International Consortium for Social Development in Kampala included "Issues of social justice and human rights" in its symposium overview. The 2014 Joint World Conference on Social Work and Social Development in Melbourne contained as one of its five themes

"Educating for change, human rights, and equality". The 2015 19th Symposium of the International Consortium for Social Development in Singapore contains the sub-theme "Human rights perspectives and human well-being". The 2016 Joint World Conference on Social Work, Education, and Social Development in Seoul also has identified human rights among its themes and topics. In addition to the prominence of human rights among the conference themes, there have also been many presentations and posters that incorporate human rights perspectives or topics delivered at these meetings.

In 2013 a special working meeting on human rights and social work was held at the University of Connecticut, organized by the School of Social Work and the Human Rights Institute. Twenty-seven social work scholars came together for two days to present working papers and discuss how to advance human rights in social work education. The conference organizers and participants developed several of these papers into an edited volume (Libal, Berthold, Thomas & Healy, 2014). Since 2012 a Special Interest Group has met at the annual Society for Social Work and Research conference in the U.S. to discuss human rights and social work; this group has also met at the Annual Program Meeting of the Council on Social Work Education (CSWE) since 2013.

Training manuals

In 1994 the UN produced the manual *Human Rights and Social Work* to raise awareness of human rights among social workers. This was in advance of the 1995 UN World Conference on Human Rights in Vienna, and the launch of the Decade of Human Rights Education. This manual, known as the *Manual for Schools of Social Work and the Social Work Profession*, stated that "More than many professions, social work educators and practitioners are conscious that their concerns are closely linked to respect for human rights . . . human rights are inseparable from social work theory, values and ethics, and practice" (UN, 1994, p. 5). In 2002 the IFSW published a training manual called *Social Work and the Rights of the Child: A Professional Training Manual on the UN Convention.*

Social work education

Recent curricula developments have seen an increase in attention to human rights within social work education. Social work education in Europe has integrated human rights content and courses to a greater degree than other regions; the only degree programs that offer social work students specialized emphasis or joint study in human rights are in Europe. The Alice Salomon Hochschule University of Applied Sciences in Berlin offers a Master of Arts in *Social Work as a Human Rights Profession*, a one-year "research-oriented, partially internet-based" study program that seeks to translate abstract human rights principles into social work practice (www.ash-berlin.eu). The program includes separate courses on human rights and social problems or vulnerable populations such as poverty and social exclusion;

culture, ethnicity, racism, and marginalization; gender; children; and health and disability. Another module includes coursework on social work practice in human rights education; within social and health agencies; at local, national, and international levels; and in public relations. The Department of Social Work at the University of Gothenburg offers a two-year master's program in *Social Work and Human Rights*. The curriculum emphasizes social work practice, service-user participation, and interdisciplinary approaches to human rights, global poverty, and international social work. The Amsterdam University of Applied Sciences' School of Social Work and Law offers a minor in *Human Rights and Civil Society* that contains several classes on human rights and social work.

Some schools of social work in the U.S. have revamped their mission and curriculum to embrace a human rights perspective in all their efforts, notably Fordham University's Graduate School of Service, the University of Buffalo's School of Social Work, and Monmouth University, often linked to trauma-informed or global perspectives.

Other schools of social work have developed specialized courses in human rights for social work students. In Europe, the social work programs that offer human rights courses include the Hague University of Applied Sciences and the University College Roosevelt in the Netherlands, Central European University in Budapest, University of Vilnius in Latvia, University of Lisbon, Portugal, and the University of Edinburgh in Scotland. In Australia, human rights and social work courses are available in the social work departments of the University of Western Sydney and Charles Sturt University. In the U.S., such courses have been offered at Silberman School of Social Work at Hunter College, University of Connecticut, University of Vermont, Smith College, University of Utah, University of Chicago, George Mason University, and Dominican University, among others.

Conversely, social work educators at Arizona State University have developed a *Social Work and Trauma* track for graduate students specializing in human rights to take social work classes as part of their two-year master's program. The University of Pennsylvania's *Global Human Rights Certificate* includes some social work courses as approved courses for law students.

The Ohio State University makes human rights advocacy a required part of social work students' fieldwork. This entails a prescribed set of hours of advocacy and 8 hours of volunteer experience during the course of students' field practicum, excepting partisan political activities, trainings, and workshops. Examples include participating in "advocacy days" and organizing and participating in letter-writing to legislators or editors.

Some schools of social work have developed study abroad trips that offer students experiences studying and learning about human rights, both explicitly and implicitly. Southern Illinois University-Carbondale offers a study abroad trip to Munich, Germany, with a specialized focus on human rights and social work. Students are introduced to human rights and European social work approaches to human rights. Florida State University offers a study abroad trip to the Czech Republic focused on social work, international affairs, and human rights. CSWE has sponsored study abroad trips for social work faculty to Costa Rica with a special emphasis upon human rights.

In the U.S., CSWE's 2008 Educational Policy Accreditation Standards (EPAS) includes as a core competency that social work education should "advance human rights and social and economic justice". The description identifies a range of human rights such as "freedom, safety, privacy, an adequate standard of living, health care, and education" which should be "distributed equitably and without prejudice". It also states that social workers should be knowledgeable of "strategies to promote human and civil rights" (CSWE, 2008, p. 3). This competency is primarily associated with advocacy practice. These standards are currently under revision; the new version will be released in 2015. The revised EPAS expands the core competency to "advance human rights and social, economic, and environmental justice". The revisions also add the language "human rights violations" after "social workers understand the global interconnections of oppression" and specify that human rights are inclusive, comprising civil, political, environmental, economic, social, and cultural rights (p. 4). The associated practice behavior is advocacy "at the individual and system levels". The 2015 EPAS also integrates human rights into policy practice and includes human rights as a core value of social work. CSWE Press has also published edited texts on integrating human rights into social work education (Hokenstad, Healy & Segal, 2013; Libal, Berthold, Thomas & Healy, 2014).

Conclusion

The growth of scholarship and education focused on human rights suggests that the field is turning towards human rights, rediscovering its rights-based roots. It is now undeniable that there is a consensus that human rights are important and relevant to social work. This review indicates that far from being an abstract or an exotic topic, human rights is and should be embedded in social work's definition, ethics, scholarship, and education. However, it may be premature to conclude that the preceding points of evidence amount to proof that social work is fully conscious of itself as a human rights-based profession; much of this signifies a rhetorical embrace. This book is an attempt to unearth the shared ground between human rights and social work and to examine the potential for human rights to enrich and empower social work by moving beyond rhetoric and into practice.

Commonalities and convergences

In addition to the ethical, educational, and scholarly developments discussed in the previous section, human rights are relevant to social work because they share many commonalities. This section reviews this common ground and makes the case that social work and human rights share common paradigms. This includes examining the overlaps in the history and development of the two fields and in their priorities towards problems requiring attention, intervention, and remediation. Additional areas of overlap such as theoretical perspectives are discussed in Chapter 2 as a means of outlining a framework for human rights-based practice. Some of the shared challenges faced by these fields as aspirational projects working to reduce human misery are discussed in Chapter 8 as conceptual and practical limitations of rights-based approaches.

History

"Social work has, from its conception, been a human rights profession" (UN, 1994, p. 3). The idea that social work is closely related to human rights, and that human rights are relevant to social work, dates to the profession's beginning (Wronka & Staub-Bernasconi, 2012). However, social work's identity as a human rights profession has been submerged, and is still not prominently recognized in many parts of the world.

Social workers were among the initial human rights leaders and active in the women's rights and suffrage movements (Healy, 2008b). Jane Addams, widely recognized as among the founding mothers of social work for her role in the settlement movement, was among the human rights pioneers of the early 20th century. Addams was a contemporary of Eleanor Roosevelt, who regarded her as among the greatest living women of the era (*New York Times*, 1935). In 1902, Addams acknowledged the human right to participation, which has the potential to "free the powers of each man and connect him with the rest of life. We ask this not merely because it is the man's right to be thus connected but because we have become convinced that the social order cannot afford to get along without his special contribution" (Addams, 1902, p. 178). Addams condemned prostitution (1912), not as immoral, but as a "global socio-economic enterprise for organized slavery" (quoted in Wronka & Staub-Bernasconi, 2012, p. 76) and linked advocacy for individual freedoms to campaigns for human rights such as the abolition of slavery in the U.S.; abolition has been referred to as the first successful global human rights campaign (Bales, 2004). Jane Addams became infamous in the U.S. for her anti-war activism. In 1915 she led the Women's Congress of The Hague in a protest against World War I, and conceptualized war itself as a human rights violation (Staub-Bernasconi, 2012). Her efforts for peace were acknowledged with the 1931 Nobel Peace Prize. Addams' social work colleagues Sophonisba Breckinridge, Julia Lathrop, and Grace Abbot were also active in the women's, children's, and labor rights movements of the early 20th century (Healy, 2008b).

The English social work pioneer Eglantine Jebb founded *Save the Children* in 1919 and drafted a *Convention of Children's Rights* in 1924 that was a precursor to the Convention on the Rights of the Child (Staub-Bernasconi, 2012). Alice Salomon, from Germany, was the founding president of IASSW and a champion of women's rights, peace, and disarmament (Healy, 2008b).

The 1947 Association of American Social Workers proposed that "all social workers should have as a major concern, those broad human rights and collective liberties that are the birthright of every individual (AASW, 1947, p. 53). Bertha Capen Reynolds in 1951 called on social work's potential to be "a profession which will stand forthrightly for human well-being, including the right to be an active citizen" (Reynolds, 1951, p. 175). The 1968 International Conference on Social Welfare focused on the theme of "social welfare and human rights" (Healy, 2008b); the president named human rights as the core professional value and named the central question for practitioners, regardless of field or specialization, as "how to implement, protect, and make real their human rights in the everyday life of people under stress" (as quoted in Staub-Bernasconi, 2012, p. 77).

Social workers have had a major impact in the development of children's rights, campaigns against apartheid and other forms of racial discrimination, and the peace movement (Albrithen & Androff, 2015; Healy, 2008b). However, most social work attention to human rights in the U.S. was subsumed in a focus on civil rights, as was the rest of the country, and only resurfaced in an episodic manner with moments such as the "welfare rights movement" (Ife, 2012).

Many of social work's contributions to human rights are unacknowledged (Healy, 2008b); even today social workers active in human rights are rarely identified as social workers. In 2003 Leymah Gbowee, a Liberian social worker, won the Nobel Peace Prize for her leadership in the women's movement against the use of rape and child soldiers in Liberia's Civil War. She has been widely identified as a women's rights activist, not as a social worker. From Jane Addams to Leymah Gbowee, social workers have made major contributions to human rights, as evidenced by their pair of Nobel Peace Prizes stretched across seven decades.

Priorities

Another area of commonality between these fields is their shared priorities. Both fields hold as their goal working towards an aspirational, utopian project. Human rights workers and social workers labor to advance human welfare with a special focus to protect and empower the weak, the poor, the vulnerable, and the oppressed. Both fields are motivated by a concern for where social problems are the "worst". This is consistent with the theory of distributive justice; that society's limited resources and capacity should be deployed in service of the disadvantaged. The union between human rights and social work is that they are both concerned with promoting people's achievement of their humanity and acknowledging the rights of disadvantaged or marginalized groups (Ife, 2012, pp. 22–23).

This priority leads to overlap in the attention given to vulnerable groups: traditional social work "client" populations and the UN's concept of vulnerable populations, which denotes people who do not have the opportunity to participate in normal community life due to social or physical barriers, often experiencing discrimination (Wronka & Staub-Bernasconi, 2012). Both fields concentrate on many of the same populations: children, the sick, the poor, the displaced, the victims, and the elderly. Both fields share a similar orientation to the problems of victims of state power (or any authoritative power), disenfranchisement, and social exclusion. This is why the topics of the core chapters in this book, despite being unusual selections for "human rights in social work" topics, are fitting choices to explore this common ground. In this way this book breaks new ground by combining the strengths of both fields.

The aim of a global human rights culture has been defined as "a lived awareness of human rights principles in one's mind and heart, and dragged into the everyday life" (Wronka & Staub-Bernasconi, 2012, p. 70). Often human rights and social work are said to be working for social justice. Social justice, however, has its limitations; it has been deemed an "important but amorphous concept" (Wronka & Staub-Bernasconi, 2012, p. 70). Others have defended the concept of social justice, and raised concerns about the loose interpretation of human rights in social work (Reisch, 2014a). Despite frequent invocations (Austin, 2013; Reisch, 2014b) social work as a profession has failed to offer or develop a coherent or meaningful definition of social justice. The U.S.'s NASW *Code of Ethics* (2008) offers only a circular statement, mandating adherence to the ethical principle of social justice by requiring that social workers engage in social justice. That is why some social work scholars have embraced human rights as a more clear and defined orientation for practice and policy. Human rights are developed and codified in international statements; this book unpacks the human rights concerns and standards across core social work fields of practice. It would appear that human rights can offer specificity, a greater public consensus, legal weight in some cases, and international credibility.

Divergences and differences

Although human rights and social work share a lot of ground as reviewed in this chapter, there are significant divergences between these fields that should not be overlooked. Despite this common ground of shared paradigms, human rights and social work are indeed separate fields. This section briefly considers the gaps between social work and human rights and provides a contrast to the previous sections by noting some important differences between the fields that will be important to consider. There is a lack of consciousness of the other on both sides. Human rights advocates, in their effort to realize human rights, identify goals that resemble social work; however, they don't know that they want to do social work and often fail to engage social work as a meaningful partner. Many human rights advocates lack social work training or any training related to the helping professions. Even while attention to human rights among social workers is growing, it has not yet permeated into the mainstream.

Social work, especially in the U.S., continues to have a narrow, perhaps uninformed, view of human rights. For example, CSWE's 2008 Education Policy and Accreditation Standards mandated that programs dealt with "human rights and civil rights", an unnecessary and confusing separation begging the difference. This false dichotomy is rampant in the U.S. and social work suffers from it too. The American Academy of Social Work and Social Welfare, as part of a Grand Challenges Initiative, has published a working paper reviewing the profession's key contributions

(Sherraden et al., 2014). While human rights is listed among social work's historical accomplishments, "human rights" is a separate entry from other rights categories, such as "women's political, civil, and human rights" (p. 6), "civil rights" (p. 7), and American Indian rights (p. 7). This reinforces the fallacy that political and civil rights are not human rights. Also, while each distinct vulnerable population does deserve its own human rights protections, splitting special populations' rights from human rights reinforces a narrow conception of human rights. Several additional entries represent achievements in children's rights (child protection) and the rights of people with mental illness (deinstitutionalization); while these developments clearly advance human rights, it is problematic that they are not identified as such even when being celebrated.

There are several reasons for this lack of consciousness that divide social work from human rights. Social work is a profession in a way that the human rights field is not. The profession of social work is comprised of social workers. One can become a social worker and find employment with this title. One can do human rights work, but usually human rights work is conducted by lawyers or other professionals. Historical analyses have traced social work's journey to professionalization, lamenting that along the way social work traded some of its justice and activist priorities in order to become institutionalized with professional credibility (Reisch & Andrews, 2001). The professional status of social work is sometimes regarded as a double-edged sword. While it helps to increase the influence and reach of social work, which ultimately increases its capacity to make a difference for the better in the world, it also should be acknowledged that professionalization has also been linked to a retreat from activism, a reluctance to engage in political activities, and a failure to challenge powerful actors in society – even when those actors are responsible for contributing to injustice, oppression, and harm.

The professionalization of social work contrasts with the activism of human rights. Human rights "workers" may be more engaged in social action, which isn't typically the primary professional activity of social work. Professional social workers are often employed by government agencies or organizations that rely on state funding. There are some activities that would compromise social workers' employment. This may contribute to a fundamental conflict of interest of the social work profession and social justice. Social workers are often "agents of the state", either employed by state agencies or government offices, or executing state policy in their practice. Human rights workers tend to be outside the system, critiquing government policy and practice, or advocating for reform. This is also a social work role as well.

In addition to being a profession, social work is a well-established academic discipline with developed educational programs and degrees. There are not departments or degrees of human rights in the same way. One can earn a degree in human rights but this is more often a specialty or interdisciplinary rather than an established academic unit. Human rights, academically and professionally, insofar as it is developed, is the purview of law and political science. The academic literature on human rights primarily consists of legal, philosophical, and political science perspectives (Ife, 2012). Although human rights are interdisciplinary, overall human rights are firmly rooted in the field of law, and widely recognized to be dominated by those from fields of law, political science, and philosophy. Human rights have been called "a legal mandate to fulfill human need" (Wronka & Staub-Bernasconi, 2012, p. 70). The disciplinary boundaries between the law and social work and related helping professions are significant, and reflect the inherent differences between law and politics, and the social work, psychology, and sociology fields. These different disciplinary perspectives reinforce the gap and reflect each field's emphasis of different methods. Human rights are focused more on rule of law and legal process than social work. Social work is more focused on mental well-being, therapeutic process, and relationships than human rights.

There is a trend toward the inclusion of more social science within human rights. One example is the use of forensic anthropology in exhumations of mass graves (Stover & Weinstein, 2004). Another is the use of statisticians in the use of documentation of human rights violations (Ball, Spirer & Spirer, 2000). Human rights have also been embraced by some medical professionals (Farmer, 2005). Without a more broad social work perspective, the purely legalistic approach to human rights limits its potential; what is legal or political is not always what is best for people's social welfare, and philosophy can be meaningless without practical application. Despite these recent extensions beyond the traditional legal framing of human rights, human rights have been underdeveloped in the social sciences. This is particularly the case with applied professions such as social work; this book is a corrective to this problem, and offers a building block to bridge the gap.

Rationale for this book

The purpose of this book is to advance the field of social work by taking the next step towards human rights. This book builds upon the previous work reviewed in this chapter that clearly links social work and human rights by continuing to reframe social work as a human rights-based profession through the articulation of rights-based approaches to social work practice. Despite the rhetorical embrace of human rights by social work, not much has been written about the application of human rights to social work practice or about the "practice of human rights" (Ife, 2012, p. 10). The status of human rights in social work "remains a 'nice idea' rather than a solid foundation for the development of practice" (Ife, 2012, p. 11). The lack of exploration in this area has muted the potential of human rights for social work.

This book aims to de-exoticize human rights for social work. Human rights in the social work literature are often treated as lofty ideals; there is a dearth of useful human rights ideas for social workers. Social workers may embrace the spirit of human rights; however, practitioners engaged in the day-to-day drudgery and gritty reality of social work practice may have skepticism about the utility of human rights. The distance between practical implementation and wishful thinking can feel insurmountable. Social work can benefit from concrete tools to assist practitioners reforming traditional practice to improve social welfare.

The core aims of this book are to enable readers to recognize and identify the linkages and interconnections between social work and human rights, to gain familiarity with the key international human rights treaties, conventions, documents, principles, standards, and guidelines that impinge upon social work, to assess social work practice from a rights-based perspective and ultimately to apply rights-based approaches to their own practice.

The global relevance of human rights

Human rights have become a priority around the world wherever people are working to promote social welfare and reduce human misery. Human rights have been called "one of the most important ideas in contemporary discourse" (Ife, 2012, p. 1). In particular, the fields of international development and global public health have made use of human rights in a way that social work has yet to do (Beyrer & Pizer, 2007; Gready & Ensor, 2005). The United Nations (UN) has embraced human rights; the UN has an Office of the High Commissioner for Human Rights, a Human Rights Council, Commission, and Center, and Working Groups and special rapporteurs on various human rights themes (Reichert, 2011, p. 207). In 2008 the UN Secretary General called for human rights to be adopted throughout the UN. Ban Ki-Moon said "There is virtually no aspect of our work that does not have a human rights dimension. Whether we are talking about peace and security, development, humanitarian action, the struggle against terrorism, climate change, none of these challenges can be addressed in isolation from human rights" (UN, 2009, p. 1). In 2009 the UN established a Human Rights Mainstreaming Mechanism (UN, 2009) to integrate rights-based approaches to all of its work. The WHO has also engaged in system-wide efforts to strengthen human rights mainstreaming at country level (WHO, 2011). The UN Office of the High Commissioner of Human Rights coordinates the UN human rights activities and works with state governments and NGOs to foster human rights (Wronka & Staub-Bernasconi, 2012). The UN has a World Program for Human Rights Education and has launched the World Decade for Human Rights Education (2005–2015) (Wronka, 2008).

In a significant way, human rights are at the center of global activity addressing core social problems. If social work is to gain greater global relevance and take its seat at the table, it will need to embrace human rights. Human rights have the potential to reinvigorate social work practice, and to advance the profession to greater global relevance. Human rights are and have been an important tool for resistance against economic globalization and the invasive, dehumanizing social forces of neo-liberalism (Ife, 2012; Lundy, 2011). Social work should not relegate human rights to the sidelines of human striving, community life, and social change processes. Social workers should not be content to permit such a valuable and powerful tool to remain inaccessible and unwieldy. Human rights should not be put in conflict with social work's priorities and preoccupations; social work's most basic elements and intractable challenges could benefit from rights-based approaches. Assessing the safety of children during a home visit, dealing with the suicidality of a client in a therapy session, having an incarcerated client, meeting the needs of children in poverty, adults with ill health, families without enough food, and communities that are excluded – these are all examples of typical social work practice situations with profound human rights implications. They echo the famous Eleanor Roosevelt quote,

> Where after all do universal human rights begin? In small places, close to home – so close and so small that they cannot be seen on any map of the world. Yet they are the world of the individual person; the neighborhood he lives in; the school or college he attends; the factory, farm or office where he works. Such are the places where every man, woman and child seeks equal justice, equal opportunity, equal dignity without discrimination. Unless these rights have meaning there, they have little meaning anywhere.
> *(Eleanor Roosevelt at the United Nations, March 27, 1958)*

Human rights can assist social work – through increased partnership, collaboration and better integration – in the realization of social justice. Integrating human rights within social work may accomplish a "double-move", simultaneously validating social work as a critically important field in the pursuit of social justice and challenging the negative aspects of social work that have perpetuated inequality, oppression, and disempowerment. Social work, in turn, can contribute to a "global human rights culture" which is often posited as an end-goal of human rights, and has been defined as "a lived awareness of human rights principles" that extend "to the feeling level, the level of the heart, and dragged into one's everyday life" (Wronka, 2008, p. 292).

Knowledge about rights-based approaches will enable social workers to become more effective advocates for social justice (Tang & Lee, 2006). In today's era of globalization, a working knowledge of human rights and how to incorporate rights into practice is virtually indispensable to contemporary activists and social change agents; human rights have become a prerequisite for practice (Tang & Lee, 2006). A better integration of human rights to social work, through examining how social workers can use human rights, can help social work become more powerful and relevant to the world.

Methodology

The methodology of this book combines a case study approach, an internationalist perspective, and a hybrid inductive and deductive approach to distill practical applications of human rights-based approaches to social work practice. This book takes five core social work domains (poverty, children, older adults, health, mental health), assesses the current state of these populations, analyzes the relevant human rights principles and standards, identifying relevant case studies, and distills rights-based approaches for social work.

This book applies an internationalist perspective (Ife, 2012) to the study of rights-based approaches to social work practice. The international perspective of this book makes the case that human rights are relevant to social workers around the globe. While there is much attention given to social work in the U.S., being where the author is situated and where social work has perhaps the most room to grow in terms of human rights, care has been taken to incorporate global perspectives and draw case studies from diverse international examples. An important caveat is that each rights-based approach must be locally contextualized to specific cultural and practice environments.

Ife (2012) identifies two approaches to human rights, the inductive and the deductive. The inductive approach to human rights entails a bottom-up approach that starts with practice experience from which it builds meaning of and for human rights. The deductive approach starts with defined human rights documents, such as the Universal Declaration or human rights conventions, and applies codified standards to specific practice situations. This book combines both. Each chapter takes the deductive approach by reviewing the international human rights documents and standards that are relevant to the chapter's practice area, and interprets what the standards mean for social work. The next section of each chapter identifies case studies from practice and examines them in light of the human rights standards as well as the framework for rights-based practice. The final section of each chapter blends the findings from the deductive and inductive sections into implications for social work practice.

References

Addams, J. (1902). *Democracy and social ethics*. New York: Macmillan.

Addams, J. (1912). *A new consciousness and an ancient evil*. New York: Macmillan.

Ainsworth, F., & Hansen, P. (2012). The experience of parents of children in care: The human rights issue. *Child & Youth Services, 32*(1), 9–18.

Albrithen, A., & Androff, D. (in press). The convergence of social work and human rights: Analyzing the historical and ethical foundations of allied disciplines. *Indian Journal of Social Work*.

Alzate, M. (2009). The role of sexual and reproductive rights in social work practice. *Affilia, 24*(2), 108–119.

American Association of Social Workers (AASW). (1947). Platform statement on international cooperation for social welfare goals, organization and principles. *Compass, 27*(4), 32–35.

Androff, D. (2010). Truth and reconciliation commissions (TRCs): An international human rights intervention and its connection to social work. *British Journal of Social Work, 40*(6), 1960–1977.

Androff, D. (2011). The problem of contemporary slavery: An international human rights challenge for social work. *International Social Work, 54*(2), 209–222.

Androff, D. (2014). Human rights and the war on immigration. In R. Furman & A. Akerman (Eds.), *Criminalization of immigration: Contexts and consequences* (pp. 147–162). Durham, NC: Carolina Academic Press.

Androff, D., Fike, C., & Rorke, J. (in press). Greening social work education: Teaching environmental rights and sustainability in community practice. *Journal of Social Work Education*.

Androff, D., & Tavassoli, K. (2012). Deaths in the desert: The human rights crisis on the US-Mexico border. *Social Work, 57*(2), 165–173.

Aotearoa New Zealand Association of Social Workers (ANZASW). (2013). *Code of Ethics*. Christchurch: Author. Retrieved from: http://anzasw.org.nz/documents/0000/0000/0664/Chapter_3_Code_of_Ethics_Summary.pdf

Asociación de Asistentes Sociales del Uruguay (ADASU). (2014). *Codigo de etica profesional del servicio social o trabajo social en el Uruguay*. Montevideo: Author. Retrieved from: www.adasu.org/prod/1/46/Codigo.de.Etica.pdf

Austin, M. (2013). *Social justice and social work: Rediscovering a core value of the profession*. Thousand Oaks, CA: Sage.

Australian Association of Social Work (AASW). (2010). *Code of Ethics*. Canberra: Author. Retrieved from: www.aasw.asn.au/document/item/1201

Ayinagadda, S. (2013). The impact of nongovernmental organizations on the promotion of child human rights in India. *Social Development Issues, 35*(2), 50–69.

Bales, K. (2004). *Disposable people: New slavery in the global economy*. Berkeley: University of California Press.

Ball, P., Spirer, H., & Spirer, L. (2000). *Making the case: Investigating large scale human rights violations using information systems and data analysis*. Washington, DC: American Association for the Advancement of Science. Retrieved from: https://hrdag.org/wp-content/uploads/2013/01/MakingtheCase-2000-intro.pdf

Berthold, M. (2015). Human rights-based approaches to clinical social work. In S. Gatenio Gabel (Ed.), *Springer briefs in rights-based approaches to social work series*. New York: Springer.

Beyrer, C., & Pizer, H. (2007). *Public health and human rights: Evidence-based approaches*. Baltimore, MD: Johns Hopkins University Press.

Briskman, L. (2006). *We've boundless plans to share: The first report of the people's inquiry into detention*. Australian Council of Heads of Schools of Social Work. Retrieved from: www.achssw.org.au/images/pdf/PIDFirstReportNov_2006Final.pdf

Briskman, L., & Cemlyn, S. (2005). Reclaiming humanity for asylum seekers: A social work response. *International Social Work, 48*(6), 714–724.

British Association of Social Work (BASW). (2012). *The Code of Ethics for Social Work: Statement of Principles*. Birmingham: Author. Retrieved from: http://cdn.basw.co.uk/upload/basw_112315-7.pdf

Bromfield, N., & Rotabi, K. (2012). Human trafficking and the Haitian child abduction attempt: Policy analysis and implications for social workers and NASW. *Journal of Social Work Values and Ethics, 9*(1), 1–25.

Buchanan, I., & Gunn, R. (2007). The interpretation of human rights in English social work: An exploration in the context of services for children and for parents with learning difficulties. *Ethics & Social Welfare, 1*(2), 147–162.

Canadian Association of Social Workers (CASW). (2005). *Code of Ethics*. Ottawa: Author. Retrieved from: http://casw-acts.ca/sites/default/files/attachements/CASW_Codeof Ethics.pdf

Cemlyn, S. (2008a). Human rights practice: possibilities and pitfalls for developing emancipatory social work. *Ethics and Social Welfare, 2*(3), 222–242.

Cemlyn, S. (2008b). Human rights and Gypsies and Travellers: An exploration of the application of human rights perspective to social work with a minority community in Britain. *British Journal of Social Work, 38*(1), 153–173.

Cemlyn, S., & Briskman, L. (2003). Asylum, children's rights and social work. *Child & Family Social Work, 8*(3), 163–178.

Chen, H., Tang, I., & Lui, P. (2013). Framing human rights and cultural diversity training in social work classrooms – the case of female marriage immigrants in Taiwan. *Affilia, 28*(4), 429–439.

Council on Social Work Education (CSWE). (2008). *Educational Policy and Accreditation Standards.* Alexandria, VA: Author. Retrieved from: www.cswe.org/File.aspx?id=41861

Cox, D., & Pawar, M. (2006). *International social work: Issues, strategies, and programs.* Thousand Oaks: Sage.

Critelli, F. (2010). Women's rights = human rights: Pakistani women against gender violence. *Journal of Sociology and Social Welfare, 37*(2), 135–160.

Dewees, M., & Roche, S. (2001). Teaching about human rights in social work. *Journal of Teaching in Social Work, 21*(1–2), 137–155.

Dominelli, L. (1998). Feminist social work: An expression of universal human rights. *Indian Journal of Social Work, 59*(4), 917.

Ellis, K. (2004). Promoting rights or avoiding litigation? The introduction of the Human Rights Act 1998 into adult social care in England. *European Journal of Social Work, 7*(3), 321–340.

Engstrom, D., & Okamura, A. (2004). A plague of our time: Torture, human rights, and social work. *Families in Society, 85*(3), 291–300.

Ericson, C. (2011). Pura Vida with a purpose: Energizing engagement with human rights through service-learning. *Advances in Social Work, 12*(1), 63–78.

Falk, D. (1999). International policy on human rights. *NASW News, 44*(3), 17.

Farmer, P. (2005). *Pathologies of power: Health, human rights, and the new war on the poor.* Berkeley: University of California Press.

Fawcett, B., & Plath, D. (2014). A national disability insurance scheme: What social work has to offer. *British Journal of Social Work, 44*(3), 747–762.

Fish, J., & Bewley, S. (2010). Using rights based approaches to conceptualise lesbian and bisexual women's health inequalities. *Health & Social Care in the Community, 18*(4), 355–362.

Gammonley, D., Rotabi, K., Forte, J., & Martin, A. (2013). Beyond study abroad: A human rights delegation to teach policy advocacy. *Journal of Social Work Education, 49*(4), 619–634.

George, J. (1999). Conceptual muddle, practical dilemma: Human rights, social development and social work education. *International Social Work, 43*(1), 15–26.

Gready, P., & Ensor, J. (Eds.). (2005). *Reinventing development: Translating rights-based approaches from theory into practice.* London: Zed Books.

Grodofsky, M. (2012). Community-based human rights advocacy practice and peace education. *International Social Work, 55*(5), 740–753.

Hagues, R. (2013). The U.S. and the Convention on the Rights of the Child: What's the hold-up? *Journal of Social Work, 13*(3), 319–324.

Harding, S., & Libal, K. (2012). Iraqi refugees and the humanitarian costs of the Iraq war: What role for social work? *International Journal of Social Welfare, 21*(1), 94–104.

Hawkins, C., & Knox, K. (2014). Educating for international social work: Human rights leadership. *International Social Work, 57*(3), 248–257.

Healy, L. (2007). Universalism and cultural relativism in social work ethics. *International Social Work, 50*(1), 11–26.

Healy, L. (2008a). *International social work: Professional action in an independent world* (2nd ed.). Oxford: Oxford University Press.

Healy, L. (2008b). Exploring the history of social work as a human rights profession. *International Social Work, 51*(6), 735–748.

Healy, L., & Kamya, H. (2014). Ethics and international discourse in social work: The case of Uganda's anti-homosexuality legislation. *Ethics & Social Welfare, 8*(2), 151–169.

Healy, L., & Link, R. (Eds.). (2012). *Handbook of international social work: Human rights, development, and the global profession.* Oxford: Oxford University Press.

Hodge, D. (2006). Advocating for the forgotten human right: Article 18 of the Universal Declaration of Human Rights – religious freedom. *International Social Work, 49*(4), 431–443.

Hodge, D. (2012). Social justice, international human rights, and religious persecution: The status of the marginalized human right – religious freedom. *Social Work & Christianity, 39*(1), 3–26.

Hokenstad, M., Healy, L., & Segal, U. (Eds.). (2013). *Teaching human rights: Curriculum resources for social work educators.* Alexandria, VA: CSWE Press.

Holscher, D., & Berhane, S. (2008). Reflections on human rights and professional solidarity: A case study of Eritrea. *International Social Work, 51*(3), 311–323.

Hounmenou, C. (2012). Monitoring human rights of persons in police lockups: Potential role of community-based organizations. *Journal of Community Practice, 20*(3), 274–292.

Ife, J. (2001). Local and global practice: Relocating social work as a human rights profession in the new global order. *European Journal of Social Work, 4*(1), 5–15.

Ife, J. (2012). *Human rights and social work: Towards rights-based practice* (3rd ed.). Cambridge: Cambridge University Press.

Ife, J., & Fiske, L. (2006). Human rights and community work: Complementary theories and practices. *International Social Work, 49*(3), 297–308.

International Association of Schools of Social Work, International Federation of Social Workers, & International Council on Social Welfare (IASWW, IFSW & ICSW). (2012). *Global Agenda for Social Work and Social Development: Commitment to Action.* Retrieved from: www.globalsocialagenda.org/

International Association of Schools of Social Work, International Federation of Social Workers, & International Council on Social Welfare (IASWW, IFSW & ICSW). (2014). *Global Definition of Social Work.* Retrieved from: http://ifsw.org/get-involved/global-definition-of-social-work/

International Federation of Social Workers (IFSW). (1988). *Policy Statement on Human Rights.* International Policy Papers. Geneva: Author.

International Federation of Social Workers (IFSW). (2002). *Social Work and the Rights of the Child: A Professional Training Manual on the UN Convention.* Berne: Author. Retrieved from: http://cdn.ifsw.org/assets/ifsw_124952–4.pdf

International Federation of Social Workers (IFSW). (2010). *Standards in Social Work Practice Meeting Human Rights.* Berlin: Author, European Region. Retrieved from: http://cdn.ifsw.org/assets/Standards_meeting_Human_Rights-_Final_Report_.pdf

International Federation of Social Workers (IFSW). (2012). *Statement of Ethical Principles.* Geneva: Author. Retrieved from: http://ifsw.org/policies/statement-of-ethical-principles/

International Federation of Social Workers & International Association of Schools of Social Work (IFSW & IASSW). (2000). *Definition of Social Work.* Geneva: Author.

Japanese Association of Certified Social Workers (JACSW). (2004). *Code of Ethics of Social Workers.* Tokyo: Author. Retrieved from: www.jacsw.or.jp/06_kokusai/IFSW/files/06_koryo_e.html

Jewell, J., Collins, K., Gargotto, L., & Dishon, A. (2009). Building the unsettling force: Social workers and the struggle for human rights. *Journal of Community Practice, 17*(3), 309–322.

Katiuzhinsky, A., & Okech, D. (2014). Human rights, cultural practices, and state policies: Implications for global social work practice and policy. *International Journal of Social Welfare, 23*(1), 80–88.

Kim, H. (2010). UN Disability Rights Convention and implications for social work practice. *Australian Social Work, 63*(1), 103–116.

Korean Association of Social Workers (KASW). (2001). *Code of Ethics*. Seoul: Author. Retrieved from: http://cdn.ifsw.org/assets/ifsw_12405–10.pdf

Korr, W., Fallon, B., & Brieland, D. (1994). UN Convention on the Rights of the Child: Implications for social work education. *International Social Work, 37*(4), 333–345.

Leslie, D. (2008). One educator's response to a gap in policy education by offering a social work course on disabilities. *Journal of Human Behavior in the Social Environment, 18*(1), 15–30.

Libal, K., Berthold, M., Thomas, R., & Healy, L. (Eds.). (2014). *Advancing human rights in social work education*. Alexandria, VA: CSWE Press.

Libal, K., & Harding, S. (2015). Human rights-based community practice in the United States. In S. Gatenio Gabel (Ed.), *Springer briefs in rights-based approaches to social work series*. New York: Springer.

Lombard, A. (2000). Enhancing a human rights culture through social work practice and training. *Social Work/Maatskaplike Werk, 36*(2), 124–140.

Lundy, C. (2011). *Social work, social justice, and human rights: A structural approach to practice* (2nd ed.). Toronto: University of Toronto Press.

Lundy, C., & van Wormer, K. (2007). Social justice, human rights, and peace: The challenge for social work in Canada and the USA. *International Social Work, 50*(6), 727–739.

Lyons, K., Hokenstad, T., Pawar, M., Huegler, N., & Hall, N. (Eds.). (2012). *The SAGE handbook of international social work*. Thousand Oaks, CA: Sage.

Mapp, S. (2014). *Human rights and social justice in a global perspective* (2nd ed.). Oxford: Oxford University Press.

Markward, M. (1999). Social development in social work practice: Enhancing human rights for children in the Czech Republic. *Social Development Issues, 21*(1), 57–61.

McPherson, J., & Abell, N. (2012). Human rights engagement and exposure: New scales to challenge social work education. *Research on Social Work Practice, 22*(6), 704–713.

Mooradian, J. (2012). Breaking the lock: Addressing 'disproportionate minority confinement' in the United States using a human rights approach. *Journal of Social Work, 12*(1), 37–50.

Morgaine, K. (2007). Domestic violence and human rights: Local challenges to a universal framework. *Journal of Sociology & Social Welfare, 34*(1), 109–129.

Nadkarni, V. (2008). Human rights perspective in social work: Illustrations from health social work. *Indian Journal of Social Work, 69*(2), 139–158.

National Association of Social Workers (NASW). (2008). *Code of Ethics*. Washington, DC: Author. Retrieved from: www.socialworkers.org/pubs/code/code.asp

New York Times. (1935, May 22). *Jane Addams, A foe of war and need*. Obituary. Retrieved from: www.nytimes.com/learning/general/onthisday/bday/0906.html

Noyoo, N. (2004). Human rights and social work in a transforming society. *International Social Work, 47*(3), 359–369.

Parker, S. (2006). International justice: the United Nations, human rights and disability. *Journal of Comparative Social Welfare, 22*(1), 63–78.

Patterson, F. (2004). Motivating students to work with elders: A strengths, social construction, and human rights and social justice approach. *Journal of Teaching in Social Work, 24*(3/4), 165–181.

Powell, F., Geoghegan, M., Scanlon, M., & Swirak, K. (2013). The Irish charity myth, child abuse and human rights: Contextualising the Ryan Report into care institutions. *British Journal of Social Work, 43*(1), 7–23.

Pyles, L. (2006). Toward a post-Katrina framework: Social work as human rights and capabilities. *Journal of Comparative Social Welfare, 22*(1), 79–88.

Reichert, E. (1998). Women's rights are human rights: Platform for action. *International Social Work, 41*(3), 371–384.

Reichert, E. (2006). *Understanding human rights: An exercise book.* Thousand Oaks, CA: Sage.

Reichert, E. (Ed). (2007). *Challenges in human rights: A social work perspective.* New York: Columbia University Press.

Reichert, E. (2011). *Social work and human rights: A foundation for policy* (2nd ed.). New York: Columbia University Press.

Reisch, M. (2014a). The boundaries of social justice: Addressing the conflict between human rights and multiculturalism in social work education. In K. Libal, M. Berthold, R. Thomas, & L. Healy (Eds.), *Advancing human rights in social work education.* Alexandria, VA: CSWE Press.

Reisch, M. (2014b). *Social policy and social justice.* Thousand Oaks, CA: Sage.

Reisch, M., & Andrews, J. (2001). *The road not taken: A history of radical social work in the United States.* New York: Brunner-Routledge.

Ren, Y., Washburn, M., & Kao, D. (2013). The role of health insurance in promoting the health equity and human rights of Chinese rural and urban children. *Social Development Issues, 35*(2), 18–34.

Reynaert, D., Bouverne-De Bie, M., & Vandevelde, S. (2010). Children's rights education and social work: Contrasting models and understanding. *International Social Work, 53*(4), 443–456.

Reynolds, B. (1951). *Social work and social living: Explorations in philosophy and practice.* New York: Citadel Press.

Rotabi, K., & Bromfield, N. (2012). The decline in intercountry adoptions and new practices of global surrogacy: Global exploitation and human rights concerns. *Affilia, 279*(2), 129–141.

Sanders, L., Martinez, R., Harner, M., Harner, M., Horner, P., & Delva, J. (2013). Grassroots responsiveness to human rights abuse: History of the Washtenaw Interfaith Coalition for Immigrant Rights. *Social Work, 58*(2), 117–125.

Secker, E. (2013). Witchcraft stigmatization in Nigeria: Challenges and successes in the implementation of child rights. *International Social Work, 56*(1), 22–36.

Sewpaul, V. (2007). Challenging East-West value dichotomies and essentializing discourse on culture and social work. *International Journal of Social Work, 16*(4), 398–407.

Sherraden, M., Stuart, P., Barth, R., Kemp, S., Lubben, J., Hawkins, J., . . . Catalano, R. (2014). *Grand accomplishments in social work.* Grand Challenges for Social Work Initiative, Working Paper No. 2. Baltimore, MD: American Academy of Social Work and Social Welfare. Retrieved from: http://aaswsw.org/wp-content/uploads/2013/12/FINAL-Grand-Accomplishments-sb-12-9-13-Final.pdf

Singapore Association of Social Workers (SASW). (1999). *Code of Professional Ethics.* Singapore: Author. Retrieved from: www.sasw.org.sg/site/about-social-work/code-of-ethics

Skegg, A. (2005). Human rights and social work: A Western imposition or empowerment to the people? *International Social Work, 48*(5), 667–672.

Solas, J. (2000). Can a radical social worker believe in human rights? *Australian Social Work, 53*(1), 65–70.

Stainton, T. (2002). Taking rights structurally: Disability, rights and social worker responses to direct payments. *British Journal of Social Work, 32*(6), 751–763.

Staub-Bernasconi, S. (2011). Human rights and social work: Philosophical and ethical reflections on a possible dialogue between East Asia and the West. *Ethics & Social Welfare, 5*(4), 331–347.

Staub-Bernasconi, S. (2012). Human rights and their relevance for social work as theory and practice. In L. Healy & R. Link (Eds.), *Handbook of international social work* (pp. 30–36). Oxford: Oxford University Press.

Steen, J. (2006). The roots of human rights advocacy and a call to action. *Social Work, 51*(2), 101–105.

Steen, J. (2012). The human rights philosophy as a values framework for the human behavior course: Integration of human rights concepts in the person-in-environment perspective. *Journal of Human Behavior in the Social Environment, 22*, 853–862.

Steen, J., & Mathiesen, S. (2005). Human rights education: Is social work behind the curve? *Journal of Teaching in Social Work, 25*(3), 143–156.

Stover, E., & Weinstein, H. (Eds.). (2004). *My neighbor, my enemy: Justice and community in the aftermath of mass atrocity.* Cambridge: Cambridge University Press.

Sulman, J., Kanee, M., Stewart, P., & Savage, D. (2007). Does difference matter? Diversity and human rights in a hospital workplace. *Social Work in Health Care, 44*(3), 145–159.

Tang, K., & Lee, J. (2006). Global social justice for older people: The case for an international convention on the rights of older people. *British Journal of Social Work, 36*(7), 1135–1150.

Townsend, P. (2006). Poverty and human rights: The role of social security and especially child benefit. *Hong Kong Journal of Social Work, 40*(1/2), 3–32.

Twill, S., & Fisher, S. (2010). Economic human rights violations experienced by women with children in the United States. *Families in Society, 91*(4), 356–362.

Union of Social Educators and Social Workers (USESW, 2003). *The Ethical Guideline of Social Educator and Social Worker.* The Russian Public Organization. Moscow: Author. Retrieved from: http://cdn.ifsw.org/assets/Russian_ethical.pdf

United Nations (UN). (1948, December 10). Universal Declaration of Human Rights. UN General Assembly. Retrieved from: www.un.org/Overview/rights.html

United Nations (UN). (1994). *Human Rights and Social Work. A Manual for Schools of Social Work and the Social Work Profession.* Professional Training Series No. 1. Geneva: Centre for Human Rights. Retrieved from: www.ohchr.org/documents/publications/training1en.pdf

United Nations (UN). (2009). *Mainstreaming Human Rights for Better Development Impact and Coherence.* New York: United Nations Development Group. Retrieved from: http://rconline.undg.org/wp-content/uploads/2011/11/HRM_2-Pager_25Oct.pdf

Van Wormer, K. (2005). Concepts for contemporary social work: Globalization, oppression, social exclusion, human rights, etc. *Social Work & Society, 3*(1), 1–10.

Van Wormer, K. (2006). *Introduction to social welfare and social work: The U.S. in global perspective.* Belmont, CA: Thomson Brooks Cole.

Van Wormer, R., & van Wormer, K. (2009). Non-abstinence-based supportive housing for persons with co-occurring disorders: A human rights perspective. *Journal of Progressive Human Services, 20*(2), 152–165.

Viviers, A., & Lombard, A. (2013). The ethics of children's participation: Fundamental to children's rights realization in Africa. *International Social Work, 56*(1), 7–21.

Watkinson, A. (2001). Advocacy tools for a global civil society. *Canadian Social Work Review, 18*(2), 267–286.

Webb, S. (2009). Against difference and diversity in social work: the case of human rights. *International Journal of Social Welfare, 18*(3), 307–316.

Williams, T., Vibbert, M., Mitchell, L., & Serwanga, R. (2009). Health and human rights of children affected by HIV/AIDS in urban Boston and rural Uganda: A cross-cultural partnership. *International Social Work, 52*(4), 539–545.

Witkin, S. (1994). A human rights approach to social work research and evaluation. *Journal of Teaching in Social Work, 8*(1–2), 239–253.

Witkin, S. (1998). Editorial: Human rights and social work. *Social Work, 43*, 197–201.

World Health Organization (WHO). (2011, December 10). *Health and Human Rights Newsletter.* No. 3. Retrieved from: www.who.int/hhr/news/newsletter_2011.pdf

Wronka, J. (2008). *Human rights and social justice: Social action and service for the helping and health professions.* Thousand Oaks, CA: Sage.

Wronka, J., & Staub-Bernasconi, S. (2012). Human rights. In K. Lyons, T. Hokenstad, M. Pawar, N. Huegler, & N. Hall (Eds.), *The SAGE handbook of international social work* (pp. 70–84). Thousand Oaks, CA: Sage.

Young, S., McKenzie, M., Schjelderup, L., & Omre, C. (2012). The rights of the child enabling community development to contribute to a valid social work practice with children at risk. *European Journal of Social Work, 15*(2), 169–184.

Yu, N. (2006). Interrogating social work: Philippine social work and human rights under martial law. *International Journal of Social Welfare, 15*(3): 257–263.

Zavirsek, D., & Herath, S. (2010). 'I want to have my future, I have a dialogue': Social work in Sri Lanka between neo-capitalism and human rights. *Social Work Education, 29*(8), 831–842.

Zorn, J. (2009). The right to stay: Challenging the policy of detention and deportation. *European Journal of Social Work, 12*(2), 247–260.

2

A FRAMEWORK FOR RIGHTS-BASED PRACTICE

What is a rights-based approach?

Before exploring rights-based approaches to specific social work fields and populations, this section considers some general comments, definitions, and meanings of rights-based approaches. The way that human rights practice has been conceptualized is primarily a means of legal practice, reflecting the prominence of the field of law. Perhaps the quintessential human rights NGO is Amnesty International, well-known for its human rights advocacy, although this is also primarily legal or political advocacy. While law is most often viewed as the main means for protecting human rights and redressing violations, this limits the potential of human rights to inform social work practice (Ife, 2012). This book aims to put social work at the center of human rights. Social work may lack the legal sophistication or philosophical nuance, but the strength of the profession is its practice and practical relevance.

Although now it has become a familiar term in the international literature, there is not a solid consensus on the definition of a "human rights-based approach" (Nyamu-Musembi & Cornwall, 2004). This reflects the reality that there is no universal recipe for rights-based approaches. Most of the definitions and descriptions of rights-based approaches employed by the UN, WHO, and major international NGOs do cover common ground; definitions of rights-based approaches prioritize the protection and promotion of human rights, the incorporation of human rights principles, the empowerment of people, and an equitable shift in power relationships (Nyamu-Musembi & Cornwall, 2004; UN, 2006). The main principles of human rights that are relevant include human dignity, nondiscrimination, transparency, accountability, and participation (UN, 2006). These five principles form the basis of the framework for a rights-based approach to social work; they are discussed in detail later in this chapter. Rights-based approaches incorporate these principles into policy, program planning, and practice (UN, 2006).

A rights-based approach to social work practice means that social work practice itself must be consistent with human rights. Social work practice must be conceived of as related to and based upon the norms of international human rights, incorporating its standards and principles. Rights-based social work practice should affirm the "whole person" by "respecting their inherent dignity, individual autonomy and independence, and their freedom to make their own choices" (Burns, 2009, p. 19). Rights-based social work practice requires new language, terminology and concepts. Rights-based social work practice means acknowledging, recognizing, and overcoming the persistent and deleterious effects of discrimination and oppression that often compromise rights and lead to poor welfare outcomes. It should also be noted that rights-based approaches entail practices that do not violate human rights. A human rights-based approach to social work is practice that puts humans first, and places humans at the center of social work (Androff, 2013).

Rights-based approaches to social work practice

Drawing from existing social work practice models

A human rights-based approach to social work draws upon mainstream social work practice theories and concepts such as the strengths perspective, respect for diversity, and cultural competence. However, a human rights-based approach to social work practice also builds upon distinct theoretical and practice traditions that have influenced contemporary social work practice. This section reviews a few of these similar models of practice to illustrate how rights-based approaches both build upon and supplement previous models, and to emphasize how rights-based approaches make a unique and new contribution to social work practice.

Human rights build upon a critical theory tradition which along with postmodernism has informed a critical social work approach to practice (Allan, Briskman & Pease, 2009; Fook, 2012). Critical social work aims to promote social justice by employing themes of discourse, subjectivity, and deconstruction to problematize oppressive social conditions, their reproduction, and the role of ideology, positivism, capitalism, and neo-liberalism. Critical social work practice consists of collective and cooperative engagement in consciousness-raising to encourage participation in transformative social change with the goal of empowerment. Critical social work has been explicitly linked to human rights (Nipperess & Briskman, 2009). Structural social work practice is another approach that influences the human rights perspective (Mullaly, 2007). Structural social work applies a Marxist analysis of capitalism, globalization, neo-conservatism, and oppression to inform social work practice so as to advance social justice and emancipation. Structural social work has also been linked to human rights (Lundy, 2011).

Both critical social work and structural social work influenced the development of anti-discriminatory social work and anti-oppressive social work practice. Anti-discriminatory social work practice addresses discrimination against individuals by institutions or systems (Okitikpi & Aymer, 2010; Thompson, 2012). The practice model focuses on identity, and prioritizes reflection upon the practitioner's positionality and privilege as sources of bias and discrimination. Anti-discriminatory practice imperatives include attending to social context, employing cultural competency, becoming an ally, and promoting social inclusion. The model of contextualizing personal experiences, beliefs, and attitudes within cultural and social groups is known as the personal–cultural–social model (Thompson, 2012). Anti-oppressive social work practice recognizes the pernicious effect of oppression across society and the structural role in social problems (Dalrymple & Burke, 2006; Dominelli, 2002). The theoretical approach seeks to integrate individual and cultural biases that generate discrimination with structural factors that maintain oppression, and the practice model aims to alleviate and prevent oppression in social structures. Special attention is paid to the power imbalance within professional practice and the care vs. control dichotomy within social work practice. Both of these models have been subject to criticism and revision (Cocker & Hafford-Letchfield, 2014).

Human rights in social work practice have similarities with other emerging practice models, such as developmental social work practice and green social work practice. Developmental social work practice involves a planned approach to social change that seeks to harmonize economic and social progress (Midgley, 2014; Midgley & Conley, 2010). This model takes a universal, population approach to progressive policies and programs including micro-enterprise, asset-building, social protection, and social investment interventions. Developmental social work practice is based on the theoretical model of social development, which has also been linked to human rights (Midgley, 2007). Green social work takes a structural approach that integrates social and physical environments and seeks to shift social work practice toward environmental justice through promoting sustainability, reducing inequalities, and combating globalization, consumption, and industrialization (Dominelli, 2012).

Key elements of rights-based approaches to social work practice

Several social work scholars have identified key elements of rights-based approaches to social work practice. Key aspects of social work practice that have been identified as synchronous with human rights are challenging oppression, empowerment, the strengths perspective, ethnic-sensitive practice, feminist practice, and cultural competence (Reichert, 2011). Human rights have been extensively linked to social justic. Human rights have been presented as a way for social work practice to prioritize social justice (Wronka, 2008) and to reclaim its social justice mission (Androff & McPherson, 2014; Wronka & Staub-Bernasconi, 2012). Human rights have been identified as a tool to advance social justice due to its normative basis in an international consensus consisting of declarations, covenants, and conventions (Gatenio Gabel, 2015). Human rights are also often linked to international social work (Healy, 2008). Human rights-based approaches to social work practice are globally focused yet domestically relevant, and offer a means to raise social work's global consciousness (Wronka & Staub-Bernasconi, 2012).

Micro practice

Human rights have been identified as being relevant to macro practice, micro practice, and a holistic, generalist practice that blends micro and macro perspectives. While most articulations of human rights in social work practice emphasize macro practice, interest has grown in exploring rights-based approaches to clinical social work practice. Human rights-based approaches to clinical practice emphasize therapeutic interventions with victims of torture, terrorism, and human trafficking, and refugees from war and mass human rights violations (Berthold, 2015). Rights-based approaches to micro practice tend to emphasize a macro component that complements clinical interventions. For example, Narrative Exposure Therapy combines individual narrative therapy with documentation of human rights violations for political and legal advocacy (McPherson, 2012).

Rights-based approaches to clinical practice center on promoting human dignity, nondiscrimination, and cultural sensitivity; the relationship between social worker and client is paramount and becomes the prime vehicle of change, education, and healing. They require equalizing the relationship between professional and client (Wronka, 2008). While professional boundaries are traditionally important to clinical practice, rights-based approaches embody a non-hierarchical approach in therapeutic work. Treating clients with respect can be critical to promoting, maintaining, or repairing someone's dignity and sense of worth and developing resilience, particularly among "at-risk" populations such as victims of discrimination, oppression, and other human rights violations (Wronka, 2008). Rights-based approaches to clinical practice thus require knowledge of human rights and focus on at-risk populations.

Macro practice

Human rights have often been linked to macro social work practice (Wronka, 2008). Human rights are conceptually universal, and have a broad appeal to macro practice fields such as policy and community practice, and macro interventions such as political and legal advocacy, consciousness-raising education campaigns, organizing, development, and research (Ife, 2012; Libal & Harding, 2015). Rights-based approaches to social work enlarge the frame of reference beyond practice with individuals and attend to preventing and resolving social problems and human rights violations among the "whole-population" (Wronka, 2008). Population-based approaches to prevention and early intervention are considered rights-based social work practice, as ensuring everyone's human rights prevents, reduces, and eliminates many social problems (Lundy, 2011; Wronka, 2008). Working for human rights involves changing structures and institutions, including the political and economic organizations of states and corporations. Human rights work has traditionally focused on governments, with their control and deployment of military and police, but also because of the state's role in the welfare among people. Rights-based approaches to macro practice also encompass the global dimension of international institutions, cooperation, and conflict; this includes multi-national and transnational corporations and institutions such as Breton Woods organizations and international development actors (Wronka, 2008).

Holistic micro and macro integration

Human rights are often associated with macro practice; however, human rights bridge micro and macro approaches as they apply simultaneously to each human and to all humans. The distinction separating levels of intervention has been criticized for limiting practitioners' scope of impact, reinforcing hierarchies and compartmentalization (Androff & McPherson, 2015; Wronka, 2008). Human rights have been presented as a means to integrate micro and macro practice (Androff & McPherson, 2015; Ife, 2012), as do generalist practice and public health interventions (Wronka, 2008). The generalist and public health model of rights-based approach to social work identifies how human rights pertain to the whole population from interpersonal, "everyday life" to global levels of intervention (Wronka, 2008). This is consistent with how critical and structural models of social work have attempted to incorporate both micro and macro practice (Ife, 2012). Rights-based approaches integrate universal and selective dimensions of policy and practice, as human rights imply universal eligibility, as well as being selective or targeted to victims of rights violations (Gatenio Gabel, 2015). An integrated generalist model of human rights-based social work practice spans personal and professional dimensions including social policy, administrative and clinical practices, and practitioners' daily lives (Wronka & Staub-Bernasconi, 2012). Rights-based approaches to social work aim to improve everyone's quality of life, and achieve what Dorothy Day called for, "a revolution of the heart" (quoted in Wronka & Staub-Bernasconi, 2012, p. 76).

Models of rights-based approaches to social work practice

A few models of rights-based approaches to social work practice have been developed.

The personal–professional model

A personal–professional model of rights-based social work practice assesses human rights violations and promotes human dignity. This model links attention to human rights from personal interactions to professional practice to form a "triple-mandate" that focuses on clients, the profession, and society (Wronka & Staub-Bernasconi, 2012). The model extends individual and structural levels of practice to professional and political advocacy to integrate the critical and radical traditions within social work to the mainstream of the profession. The importance of human relationships is emphasized and economic, social and cultural rights are prioritized. Practice roles for social workers include empowerment of vulnerable people; advocacy with and on behalf of those who can't speak for themselves; capability-training through education, mediation, leveraging resources, and disseminating information; and public consciousness-raising about human rights issues, organizations, and mechanisms. Wronka and Staub-Bernasconi (2012) argue that such a model could avoid Western colonialism in the pursuit of universal rights. Effective preparation of practitioners in this model requires the inclusion of human rights into social work education, not as an add-on to existing curricula, but full integration in order to build a human rights culture in social work.

Three generation practice model

Although Ife (2012) refrains from specific practice prescriptions as anathema to the spirit of human rights, and is critical in general of the three generations schema, he has developed a model of practice that integrates the three generations of human rights. Micro and macro practice roles are seen as necessary to protect all rights and therefore applicable to each generation of practice. First generation human rights, civil and political rights, form the basis for social work advocacy which focuses upon victims of state violence and oppression. First generation rights links together social work practice areas in political advocacy, refugees and immigrants, forensic social work, prison reform, access to legal representation, and collaboration with lawyers. The emphasis is upon advocacy methods, where social work expertise in objective evaluation and assessment may actually hinder practice, in contrast with legal training that prepares practitioners to take advocacy positions in adversarial systems.

Second generation human rights, economic, social, and cultural rights, form the basis for social work practice in the areas of direct services; organizational, administrative, or managerial practice; policy practice and social action; and research. Second generation rights involve adequate standards of living, health, housing, and education that require the provision of social services by social work practitioners, agencies, and organizations. This set of rights is the most clearly connected with traditional social work practice to ensure social welfare, and the human rights area with which social work is most often identified. Second generation rights are also called positive rights, meaning their provision requires public expenditure, which is why this generation of rights is linked to political engagement through policy practice and social action to fund the direct services required for meeting second generation rights.

Third generation rights, collective rights such as the right to development, clean water, and peace, form the basis for social work practice geared toward community development. Community development to realize collective rights spans six dimensions: social development for strengthening social structures, cohesion, and interaction; sustainable economic development; political development focusing on decision making and power structures; cultural development for attending to communities' identity, history, traditions, values, and norms; environmental development emphasizing the physical and built environment as well as sustainability; and personal or spiritual development including personal growth, fulfillment, and individual and collective spirituality or religion. Community development for realizing collective rights should holistically integrate these dimensions.

Human rights practice in social work

Perhaps the most developed model is comprised of pillars and components of practice that attend to process and outcomes (McPherson, 2015). Pillars refer to practice based upon a human rights perspective and rights-based tools and strategies. The three pillars include a human rights lens, human rights methods, and human rights goals. These three pillars of practice represent three tiers, and each one has different components of practice. The first tier, a human rights lens, includes three components of practice that re-conceive clients as rights-holders, needs as lack of access to rights, and social problems as human rights violations. The second tier, human rights methods, has eight components of practice that include participation, non-discrimination, strengths-perspective, micro/macro integration, capacity-building, community and interdisciplinary collaboration, activism, and accountability. The third tier, human rights goals, includes two components of practice: human rights assessment and human rights goal-settings.

Conclusion

This review demonstrates the congruence of many traditional models of social work practice with human rights, and identifies aspects of rights-based approaches to social work practice, including initial steps that have been made toward developing a rights-based approach to social work practice. These models tie human rights to aspects of social work practice. While each of these approaches has merit, none have articulated specific practice guidelines or implications for applying human rights principles to practice behaviors.

The three generations model of social work practice demonstrates that social work practice can be relevant to the full range of all three generations of rights. However, as Ife (2012) notes, the three generations formulation of human rights is problematic, and thus its application to social work practice. While the three generations formulation is historically and politically significant, in actual practice it is an artificial division. To base practice upon the distinction of three generations is unnecessarily confusing; in fact the first and second generations of practice illuminate the conceptual problems with the three generations of human rights. First generation practice of political and civil advocacy blurs with the second generation of rights in terms of direct treatment for survivors and victims of violence; the second generation of practice includes policy practice and social action – both of which are powerful forms of advocacy. Ife (2012) raises the point that second generation rights are positive rights and therefore require funding; however, this commonly made point about second generation rights fails to recognize the expenditure required to provide and protect first generation rights, such as the funding necessary for a functioning legal system and law enforcement. This model de-emphasizes research and social action, which although linked to second generation can and should apply to all human rights and levels of practice, especially political and collective rights. In reality, multiple forms of social work practice relate to various generations of rights.

The question remains, what does a human rights-based social work practice look like? The answer requires a more fully defined theoretical practice framework. This is developed in the second half of this chapter. The remainder of the book grounds this theoretical framework in practice through case studies that respond to aspirational international human rights standards, enabling social work to have a greater relevance in human rights, and accommodate rights-based approaches to all dimensions and areas of social work.

A new framework for rights-based social work practice

This section presents a theoretical framework for rights-based practice. This framework applies across levels of social work practice; this is consistent with the generalist and micro/macro integration perspectives on rights-based social work discussed above. Thus this framework is based on the assumption that rights-based approaches to social work apply to both clinically oriented as well as community, organization, and policy oriented social work practice. Human rights-based approaches have the potential to influence all areas of social work practice. They should not be linked only to macro practice; this field is already marginalized within social work (Rothman & Mizrahi, 2014). This framework puts human rights at the center of social work, and this should prevent human rights from becoming "simply a field in which some advocacy-based social workers specialise" (Ife, 2012, p. 43).

Human rights provide the framework that guides policy and practice interventions. Rights-based approaches to social work put tools into the hands of practitioners who are engaged in the muddy work of transforming human misery into its highest potentials of freedom, compassion, and healing. Rights-based approaches to social work practice build upon and deepen the relational context of social work. Social work is fundamentally about human relationships. From the ethical principle of the "importance of human relationships" (NASW, 2008) to the practice techniques of "the therapeutic use of self" to the defining theoretical construct of "persons-in-environment" – social work is fundamentally about people, about people working together, and about understanding people in their varying contexts, and working to improve such contexts that affect people's well-being. The human rights conception also sets out a fundamental relationship, the relationship between rights-holders and duty-bearers. A rights-holder is entitled to rights which a duty-bearer is obligated to respect. Informed by human rights principles, rights-based practice is about developing the capacity of duty-bearers to meet their obligations, and empowering rights-holders to effectively claim their rights.

Principles of rights-based social work practice

Human rights principles have been identified that can be incorporated into social work practice (Gatenio Gabel, 2015). These principles are nondiscrimination, participation, transparency, and accountability (Baderin & McCorquodale, 2007). "Rights-based", in this sense, refers to these principles as enshrined in international human rights standards. Incorporating human rights principles into social work practice prioritizes both process and outcome. The basis of practice should shift away from human needs to human rights in order to promote human dignity, and emphasizes incorporating client populations' active participation in decision-making processes to ensure that their interests are served (Gatenio Gabel, 2015). This model of practice is seen as dynamic, as people's consensus on rights are continually re-evaluated and the understanding of rights continues to evolve; therefore new approaches to human rights in social work practice will continue to develop.

These principles form the basis for the framework of rights-based social work practice used in this book. Rights-based social work should also promote human dignity, which is an undercurrent through these four principles and yet a foundational value for all of them as well as social work. Taken together, the human rights principles of dignity, nondiscrimination, participation, transparency, and accountability encapsulate a paradigm shift from traditional social work services towards rights-based approaches.

These principles rest upon the assumption that all human rights are universal and inalienable, that everyone is a rights-holder, that no one can take another's rights away from them, and that every state has the responsibility to respect and protect human rights. They are also assumed to be indivisible, interdependent, and interrelated, meaning that all rights are equal and cannot be ranked or prioritized.

The five principles of the framework are represented as a wheel in the diagram below (Figure 2.1). These have been identified as core human rights principles as well as social work values (Albrithen & Androff, 2015). The rest of the chapter discusses each principle for practice in turn.

Human dignity

The first principle of rights-based social work practice is human dignity, also referred to as dignity and worth of the person. The principle of dignity in practice means that people are identified as rights-holders, and that the basis of practice becomes human rights, rather than human needs. This involves the incorporation of new language, as clients and consumers become rights-holders. The rights-based principle of dignity means shifting focus from needs to rights, and reconceptualizing people as rights-holders rather than clients or consumers (Gatenio Gabel, 2015). Respect for human dignity is the basis for all human rights. Human dignity is the linchpin of the rights-based practice framework, and the central link between human rights and social work. It is the principle that connects many aspects of the framework:

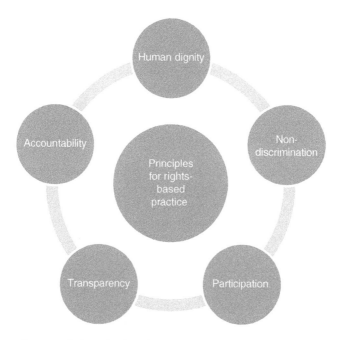

FIGURE 2.1   Framework for rights-based practice

moving from needs to rights affords more dignity as it moves people from being needy to being rights-holders. Non-hierarchical approaches also promote dignity by avoiding the denigrating or disempowering effects of hierarchical relationships.

Dignity means respect. Dignity is a core aspect of social work ethics, and fundamental to human rights. Article 1 of the UDHR (UN, 1948) states that "all humans are born free and equal in dignity and rights". The *Global Agenda* lists "Promoting the dignity and worth of peoples" as one of its core pillars (IASSW, IFSW & ICSW, 2012). The NASW *Code of Ethics* (2008) names one of the core ethical principles guiding the social work profession to be that "social workers respect the inherent dignity and worth of the person". The *Code of Ethics* goes on to relate this principle to non-discrimination, self-determination, diversity, empowerment, and the profession's dual responsibility to clients and to society.

Embedded in the principle of dignity is the concept of self-determination, which means that people should have the freedom of choice (Gatenio Gabel, 2015). Self-determination is a social work ethical value and human rights concept (Reichert, 2011). In addition to being a central feature of social work practice, in that practitioners must always respect the rights-holder's wishes concerning interventions, self-determination is also a core value of democracy, as a political science, international relations, and rule of law concept. The NASW *Code of Ethics* (2008) lists self-determination as one of the core ethical responsibilities of social workers to clients. Social workers' ethical responsibilities to society include expanding "choice and opportunity for all people".

A main benefit of placing dignity at the front of rights-based practice, and of consciously shifting the focus of practice from needs to rights, is to combat dehumanization and to promote humanization. Dehumanization has been linked to human rights violations. While helping to ensure that people's needs are met does speak to their dignity, reframing their "neediness" and dependency into a something to which they are entitled is more humanizing. Casting clients as needy at some level dehumanizes them as "less-than" and therefore diminished; this is especially so when their perceived or labeled neediness creates or reinforces stigma and discrimination.

The rights-based principle for practice of human dignity requires a shift of focus from human needs to human rights (Wronka, 2008). This is how the principle of human dignity promotes respect and the inherent worth of the person. A rights-based approach, in the principle of dignity, avoids charity (Gatenio Gabel, 2015). As Nelson Mandela said, "overcoming poverty is not a task of charity, it is an act of justice" (Mandela, 2005). This principle re-imagines the basis of social allocation, or eligibility, for social work practice. A need-based understanding of eligibility only allocates a social good to those in need, however defined and measured. This carries with it stigma. It is typically implemented in social policy by social allocation on the basis of selective eligibility, sometimes by means-testing. By contrast a rights-based understanding of eligibility is universal and applies to everyone. The framework element of dignity involves reconceptualizing "eligibility". These rights-based principles mean that the basis of social allocation should become universal rather than selective, on the basis of their humanity (Gilbert & Terrell, 2012). Eligibility in terms of access to practice and programs, and the basis of social allocation in terms of policy benefits, social goods, and public resources, should be open to all "whose quality of life is imminently threatened by denial of human rights" (Wronka, 2008, p. 157).

Macro approaches that attend to the whole population do not focus on a *needs* basis. Ife (2012) writes that some have criticized the needs preoccupation of social workers as "society's professional needs-definers". When the professional expertise is required to identify and define a need, people become disempowered as their ability to define and communicate their own need is stripped from them; people become dependent upon practitioners to define their needs for them. Needs, as a basis for social work practice, have been criticized from a human rights perspective (Gatenio Gabel, 2015). These can be understood as promoting dignity and reducing stigma. Macro level interventions and approaches that address a whole population can be categorized as "primary prevention" (Wronka, 2008). Therefore prevention programs can be considered approaches that focus on an aspect of human rights rather than needs. Prevention isn't need based. Primary prevention, public health, and whole-population approaches do not design or target interventions based on an expressed need or "pathology". Instead these approaches seek to preempt the onset of need, illness, or pathology and to do so for everyone. In the same way, the principle of dignity also informs interventions for sustainability that focus on the long-term success of individuals, families and communities. However, it should be noted that from a policy perspective, rights-based approaches can also be selective in addition to universal, insofar as they are targeted to the victims of human rights violations.

The IFSW statement on Human Rights and Extreme Poverty explains the connection between human needs and human rights by stating that "Human rights constitute the legal mandate to fulfill human needs" (Wronka, 2008, p. 137). In this way, needs and rights are seen as interdependent mirrors of each other. The concept of human needs is that to appropriately respond to a need, one must assess, evaluate, measure, characterize, and quantify that need. These processes are subject to debate. Accurate information about the nature and extent of human need will always be short. In reality, all humans have needs, and certain aspects of human needs are universal. Needs can be categorized as spiritual, cognitive, physical, and self-actualization (Wronka, 2008): the spiritual need to be treated with dignity and respect; the cognitive need for expression, information, and to be free from fear; the physical need to sustenance; the social need for belonging and community; and the self-actualization need for learning, growth, and for developing and reaching one's potential.

In practice, dignity means incorporating new language such as "rights-holders", incorporating universality as the basis for social allocation, respecting self-determination, respecting the inherent worth of every person, and employing the strength perspective (McPherson, 2015; Wronka & Staub-Bernasconi, 2012). It is about asking and answering: how can rights-based approaches to social work practice ensure that people have dignity in their everyday lives?

Nondiscrimination

The second principle of the rights-based framework is nondiscrimination. Non-discrimination is a principle that speaks to the universality of human rights; it is a fundamental human rights principle. Nondiscrimination is also a social work priority, as the *Code of Ethics* has that language about applying to everyone regardless of race, religion, ethnicity, etc. The dignity and worth of persons implies nondiscrimination (Wronka, 2008). Article 2 of the UDHR prohibits discrimination on the specific grounds of "race, color, sex, language, religion, political or other opinion, national or social origin, property, birth or other status". This has been expanded to include sexual orientation, age, ability status, and more. This is the principle that dictates that human rights apply to everyone, to every human, regardless of status or any category. These categories are listed in human rights documents and they continue to evolve. This is evidenced by the male-dominant, gendered language of the *Universal Declaration* (UN, 1948). Social work prohibits discrimination, and the *Code of Ethics* says that social workers are ethically responsible for preventing and eliminating discrimination "against any person, group or class on the basis of race, ethnicity, national origin, color, sex, sexual orientation, gender identity or expression, age, marital status, political belief, religion, immigration status, or mental or physical disability".

This means practice that is inclusive and non-hierarchical, and that incorporates cultural competence and respect for diversity (McPherson, 2015). Human rights are important to helping those who suffer discrimination. This human rights principle promotes inclusivity which is both a social work perspective and even a practice principle for community work and macro practice. In social work macro practice such as community practice, in models such as coalition building, social movements, and local organizing, the practice is to include everyone to build engagement, encouraging the investment of stakeholders. This is basic community organizing because getting people engaged and demonstrating, convincing, and communicating how it can be in people's best interest to participate is a key factor in building successful movements and organizations. This also relates to the principle of participation, as all these are overlapping.

The principle of nondiscrimination for rights-based social work practice means attending to historically disadvantaged and vulnerable populations. Nondiscrimination, in terms of being inclusive of everyone, means including those who have been previously excluded, and faced historical and current discrimination. This carries forth the principles of cultural competence and respect for diversity. Nondiscrimination in practice should prevent disparities in diagnosis among racial and other lines (Wronka, 2008). Important human rights concepts include universality and indivisibility. Indivisibility is similar to the social work concept of intersectionality of oppression. Indivisibility also means that states or groups or anyone can't prioritize certain human rights over others. For example, the Millennium Development Goals are also indivisible, and an acknowledgment that rights can't be compartmentalized.

Cultural competence relates to this as well because it involves clients maintaining respect for clients' differences, and effective practice with diversity. The strengths perspective is also relevant here because, especially when working with marginalized, vulnerable populations who are often victims of discrimination, it emphasizes the positive aspects of groups that are traditional victims of discrimination.

Nondiscrimination in social work practice means several things. Rights-based social work practice based on nondiscrimination means ensuring access to professionals, services, and resources for all people, including marginalized and underserved populations. In addition it means selective targeting of minorities, attending to the special needs of highly vulnerable groups in order to work to end disparities. This entails promoting and respecting diversity and cultural competence.

Cultural competence, as a concept for rights-based practice, is a loose term that incorporates multicultural competence and indigenous social work practice. Cultural competence is defined in the CSWE *Education Policy and Accreditation Standards* as a mindset of social work practitioners in which they view themselves as a learner, and the consumer as a teacher (CSWE, 2008). Drawing upon a Freirean approach, social workers are to engage with those they help as "informants" (CSWE, 2008). Respect for other cultures, diversity, and difference is key for practitioners, as is understanding one's own cultural background and its influence in one's own perceptions. Cultural competence is definitely not about learning a list of characteristics about a culture – that approach can lead to stereotypes, generalizations, and a closed mind. Social work was born in part through efforts to help populations that are different from the mainstream, such as migrant workers in urban industrial centers in the late 19th century. The NASW *Code of Ethics* states: "social workers are sensitive to cultural and ethnic diversity and strive to end discrimination, oppression, poverty, and other forms of social injustice" (NASW, 2008). The CSWE 2008 *Education Policy and Accreditation Standards* highlight the importance of respect for diversity. "Social workers understand how diversity characterizes and shapes the human experience . . . the dimensions of diversity are understood as the intersectionality of multiple factors including age, class, color, culture, disability, ethnicity, gender, gender identity and expression, immigration status, political ideology, race, religion, sex, and sexual orientation" (p. 5). Nondiscrimination also means displaying cultural sensitivity. Cultural sensitivity means to not base interventions or treatment on nonconformity to social or cultural norms, and to adapt interventions and treatments as well as professional communication, as best as possible, to the persons' or communities' cultural background (Wronka, 2008).

In addition to inclusivity, the principle of nondiscrimination in rights-based social work practice means dissolving hierarchies between professional workers and clients. Nondiscrimination also implies non-hierarchical approaches. "A non-hierarchical approach to helping" is one of the principles for a human rights approach to helping, or to clinical practice, or to working with "at-risk" populations (Wronka, 2008, p. 106). For professional practice, this means evening or reducing the power differential between social workers and their clients. CSWE (2011) notes some research that indicates that social workers (based on self-report) are more likely to treat clients as equals when it comes to service planning (Hardiman & Hodges, 2008). However there are numerous accounts (CSWE, 2011) of social workers adhering to traditional models of social work practice which are based upon the establishment and maintenance of a power differential between the professional and the client. Such power differentials are based inherently in the dynamic of helper and help-seeker, but in the social work context they are reinforced by additional elements of graduate education, formalized training, and advanced specialized techniques. Also variables such as the office logistics (scheduling location and pay) play a role. The mixed legacy of professionalization must also be acknowledged.

Hierarchy in helping is bad because it reinforces the original condition and status that put the receiver in a position to be helped. Hierarchy neglects the interdependence between all people. Part of the problem with professionalization and hierarchical helping relationships is the potential for the abuse of power in terms of exploitation, discrimination or stigmatization, disempowerment, and reinforcement of oppression (Wronka, 2008). As seen with "social work's shadow side", helpers – especially but not exclusively professional helpers – can perpetrate abuses in the name of helping others and even harm those they are trying to help without intending to, but by virtue of participating in hierarchical and disempowering arrangements.

This draws on the critical tradition of Paulo Freire and relies upon the common humanity of both practitioners and those they seek to help. It also recognizes the humanity of practitioners, who also enjoy the same human rights of their so-called clients. Dissolving hierarchies means transcending professionalism (Wronka, 2008).

In some cases of cross-cultural work, such as indigenization approaches to social work diffusion, social work practice has to be made less formal, and should in fact be more informal, in order to adapt to a new culture (Nimmagadda & Martell, 2008). There are examples of when undue emphasis upon the trappings of professionalism constructs an artificial barrier between practitioners and people. Indigenous social work or what has been called home-made social work, can involve bending or breaking some of the rules of professionalization, in order to maximize impact of practice. This echoes some of the critiques of professionalization, which, although it may have strengthened the stability of social work practice, has also eroded its ability and efficacy at addressing social justice.

The concept of meta-micro refers to the healing and redemptive power of everyday life (Wronka, 2008). It helps to acknowledge that professionals do not have a monopoly on helping, health, and healing (Wronka, 2008). Keeping a strengths-based perspective aids social workers to recognize everyone's potential for offering healing to others. Everyday life may seem outside of the scope of social work practice, but it is arguably the most important factor in people's well-being – their daily activities, interactions with family and friends, intimate relationships, and coping with everyday struggles – even interactions with strangers. This concept of the meta-micro (Wronka, 2008), the transformative power that exists inside every human interaction, is best accessed by practitioners able and willing to let down their professional facades a little bit. Or put another way, to "transcend" their professional boundaries to "relate to humans as other human beings". This is also the essence of Freire's view of working with the oppressed, of standing with love in solidarity with the oppressed. Working in solidarity with others is part of the foundation of empowerment. As the Aboriginal saying goes, "if you have come here to help me, you are wasting your time. But if you have come because your liberation is bound up with mine, then let us work together", often credited to an Aboriginal social worker (Aboriginal activists group, Queensland, 1970s). The question becomes how can we promote human rights in everyday life? What can rights-based approaches to social work practice do to prevent discrimination?

A nonhierarchical approach would mean a more concentric, free-flowing, horizontal, and expansive practice (Wronka, 2008). Nondiscrimination – this principle, applied to practice, means avoiding labeling and the harm to clients that comes from labeling, such as stigma and discrimination (Wronka, 2008). Practitioners should be especially aware of issues of disparities and disproportionalities. By taking a nondiscriminatory approach to practice, they can avoid diagnosing on the basis of race, ethnicity, class, religion, or other group. Nonhierarchy in practice means not framing clients as disempowered subjects, with disorders and little agency (Wronka, 2008). It also means recognizing the disempowering implications of "interventions" as something that a professional does to a client.

Participation

The third element of the framework is participation. Participation is a fundamental human rights principle as well as an important social work priority. Participation is both a human right, and a means to access or secure other human rights (Pells, 2010). Gatenio Gabel (2015) writes that the participation of all people in decision making, especially those people affected by such decisions, is a key aspect of rights-based approaches to social work practice. "Nothing about us, without us" is an expression of the central rights-based principle of participation, a slogan made famous by the disability rights movement. Participation is related to the ethical principle of social justice, which states that social workers should strive to ensure "meaningful participation in decision making for all people". The *Code of Ethics* mandates social workers' ethical responsibilities to the broader society to include public participation, through the facilitation of "informed participation by the public in shaping social policies and institutions" (NASW, 2008).

The principle of participation seeks to incorporate the voices of service-users into services, programs, and policies (Wronka, 2008). This entails a collaborative process with service-users, raising and lifting their voices, asking and incorporating the views of service-users, and ensuring informed consent, which means making sure that people can meaningfully participate in their treatment. Participation in social work practice draws upon empowerment and social pedagogy models pioneered by Paulo Freire (2000). This draws heavily from community practice which encompasses recruiting community members into social movements and community organizing efforts, as well as other macro practice methods that seek to involve service-users into program planning, evaluation, and policy design (McPherson, 2015). Other notable interventions for rights-based participation are the *promotora* model and participatory research. Interventions that foster democratic processes are also important, including recent developments in participatory budgeting.

At its core, human rights, and rights-based approaches, are about altering the relations of power, to borrow a term from community organizing, in order to equalize the distribution of power. Human rights also seek to give people access, opportunity, and ability to exercise power within and between societies. Special attention is given to mitigating the powerlessness of vulnerable populations. This necessitates the active and informed participation of people in the formulation, implementation, and monitoring of rights-based approaches. Frederick Douglass said that "power concedes nothing without a demand", and participation is the primary method for organizing people to make such demands. However, participation has also become a buzzword and caution must be given to ensuring meaningful, not token participation (Cornwall, 2008).

For participation to be meaningful, people must have the skills necessary for effective action. This often requires building the capacity of people and groups to engage in organized strategic action. Capacity building is a rights-based approach that connects interwoven systems of rights and obligations of states, international actors, and individuals. Capacities include skills, abilities, resources, responsibilities, authority, and motivation. This rights-based capacity development builds both duty-bearers' capacity for accountability and rights-holders' capacity for empowerment. As duty-bearers fulfill their obligations and rights-holders claim and exercise the enjoyment of their rights, together they achieve the realization of human rights.

Transparency

The fourth rights-based principle for social work practice is transparency. Transparency generally refers to clarity and access to information, especially as it pertains to those in power, such as transparency in decision making, in policy, and in budgets. Transparency as a human rights principle also means anti-corruption. Corruption in government is conceived as a spectrum with corruption on the negative pole, and transparency on the positive pole. This is exemplified by the well-known anti-corruption NGO Transparency International (www.transparency.org).

Rights-based approaches apply transparency to practice in the area of assessment. Assessment is a tool for seeing clearly, or transparently. Transparency, as a human rights concept applied to assessment, means incorporating human rights into assessment. Assessment is a fundamental aspect of social work practice. Assessment is vital to rights-based social work when it includes assessing human rights violations as a diagnostic category (Wronka & Staub-Bernasconi, 2012). However, assessment and diagnosis must be prevented from becoming labeling and reinforcing stigmatization (Wronka, 2008).

Transparency refers to violations of rights and to the responsibility to protect rights. Transparency in the assessment of violations, and responsibility requires taking a systems-oriented perspective (Wronka, 2008). This should happen in the assessment of human rights violations as an additional diagnostic category (Wronka & Staub-Bernasconi, 2012) and in the assessment of the responsibility to protect the human rights that are found to be violated (Jones, 2005). Assessing human rights violations in social work practice is especially important in the assessment of violations of economic, social, and cultural rights – which are more often neglected in the realm of international NGO advocacy than civil and political rights.

The responsibilities that accompany human rights encompass many systems, including national governments (Huenchuan & Rodriguez-Pinero, 2011). States, as the entities that participate in international human rights agreements and powerful actors in the welfare of their people, bear primary responsibility for protecting human rights. However, human rights are everyone's responsibility, including institutions, companies, organizations, and communities. State responsibilities include duties or obligations, such as non-interference, protection, and promotion. Non-interference means that states must avoid violating human rights, and not prevent people from enjoying their rights. Protection means that states must protect people's rights against interference by third parties that would violate or prevent the realization of human rights. Promotion means that states have an affirmative duty to provide for the realization of rights. Each of these obligations can be subjects of rights-based assessment.

The UN and human rights NGOs have developed a three-step problem analysis for assessing violations of human rights: analysis of cause, role, and capacity (Jones, 2005). First the causal analysis assesses if a human right has been violated and if so, which right. Second, the role analysis assesses which duty-bearer has the responsibility to protect the right that has been violated. Third, the capacity gap analysis assesses what is required, and what capacity or capability could be developed, to rectify the violation and restore the rights-holder. This type of assessment can be refined and extended for use in social work practice. Assessment scales could be further developed that distinguish between minor, middle, and grave violations. Assessments should be a tool to guide practitioners and result in greater transparency, not in reductionist understandings of human behavior.

Social work practice can also apply the principle of transparency when it utilizes human rights monitoring and reporting mechanisms to bring awareness and clarity to human rights violations. The UN High Commission on Human Rights and the Human Rights Council have special procedures to monitor, examine, and publicly report on specific human rights issues of concern, or human rights situations in specific countries, or global human rights themes (UN, 2001). Transparency in rights-based practice involves integrating micro and macro levels of practice, interdisciplinary collaboration, activism and accountability (McPherson, 2015).

Finally, transparency in social work practice is necessary for ensuring that social work practice does not violate human rights. Transparency is a principle that should be applied to social work policies, programs, education, research, and practitioners. When social work practice is transparent, violations of human rights in the name of helping others can be stopped and prevented.

Accountability

The fifth and final element of the framework is accountability. Accountability naturally follows transparency. Having assessed human rights violations, then determined the responsible party, an action or intervention plan can be developed to hold people accountable for their actions and to work to prevent future violations and strengthen protections. The principle of accountability is linked to the practice of advocacy. Advocacy is necessary for rights-based social work practice (UN, 1994). Advocacy can also relate to participation; social workers should engage in advocacy *with* victims of rights violations and focus on building people's capacity to raise their voices and speak for themselves (Ife, 2012). Rights-based social work practice means employing strategies and using interventions to hold actors accountable for violations of human rights. Such actors may be people, institutions, organizations, or states. Most traditional human rights campaigns and approaches would fall into what social workers would categorize as macro practice. Certainly human rights-based approaches are consistent with macro practice, especially the central pillars of community and policy practice.

Advocacy strategies that are well established in human rights, and can be incorporated into social work practice, include the naming and shaming of perpetrators of human rights violations, lobbying and pressuring states on behalf of human rights issues, deploying media tactics, conducting education and awareness raising campaigns, generating publicity and popular support, organizing, letter writing campaigns, and organizing local human rights groups such as campus chapters of Amnesty International. Legal advocacy should also be considered an important strategy for promoting accountability for human rights (Ezell, 2001; Midgley, 2007). Amnesty International is a good example of this type of macro approach, for example in their Global Campaign for Human Dignity, which focuses on economic, social, and cultural rights (Wronka, 2008).

Rights-based approaches to accountability should also make use of advocacy at the UN and through other international human rights mechanisms. In addition to promoting transparency through its monitoring reports, the UN Human Rights Council also promotes accountability by taking human rights complaints in an individual confidential 1503 complaints procedure, after domestic remedies have been exhausted. Several treaty bodies have individual complaint mechanisms where victims of human rights violations submit cases directly to committees monitoring implementation of covenants and conventions. An Optional Protocol for the International Covenant on Economic, Social and Cultural Rights created an individual complaint mechanism for economic, social, and cultural rights which entered into force in 2013. Additional treaty bodies that allow for individual complaint mechanisms include the Committee against Torture, the Committee on the Elimination of Racial Discrimination, the Committee on the Elimination of Discrimination against Women, and the Committee on Migrant Workers. Two more committees, the Committee on the Rights of Persons with Disabilities, and the Committee on Enforced Disappearances, will be created when their conventions enter into force, upon receiving 10 signatories. Special rapporteurs can also receive complaints from individuals or NGOs. After reviewing complaints and determining them to be serious and credible, treaty bodies release findings and recommendations to the appropriate responsible party or duty-bearer.

Treaty bodies monitor the adherence of state parties through the review of regular reports submitted by state parties, UN agencies, and civil society organizations. Non-state reports are sometimes called shadow or parallel reports. After reviewing state and shadow reports, the treaty body engages in a process of constructive dialogue with the state party over human rights issues (UN, 2008). Shadow reports are another avenue where social workers can advocate for human rights at the Human Rights Council or treaty bodies (Wronka & Staub-Bernasconi, 2012). The Human Rights Council conducts Universal Periodic Reviews of individual state human rights protections and violations; these reviews offer additional opportunities for social workers to advocate for human rights. Social work professional bodies such as the IASSW, among other NGOs, regularly consult with the Human Rights Council in open dialogue sessions and through position statements on global social welfare issues. Social workers can work with their professional organizations that consult at the Council and other treaty bodies. Professional organizations are also important sites for accountability in the development and implementation of ethical codes of practice. Social workers should ensure that ethical codes of conduct for practitioners are consistent with human rights, and then work to hold practitioners accountable to these codes (Wronka, 2008).

An integrative framework of first, second, and third generation rights

This framework is an integrative model for rights-based approaches to social work practice. The three generations schema of human rights has practical uses despite its flaws. It is quick, easy, makes sense, and maps onto important historical, geopolitical, and ideological points of reference.

First generation human rights correlate with the Western region of liberal, capitalist democracies that prioritize civil and political rights, primarily from an individual perspective, including free speech, freedom of religion, the right to free assembly, rights to life, privacy, non-interference from the state, due process, equal protection, freedom from torture, detention, and killing. However, the first generation of civil and political rights is an extremely limited conceptualization. The concept of rights has evolved from a more narrow view of civil rights over half a century ago, to human rights today (Wronka, 2008). Even civil rights leaders were clear about placing the civil rights movement within the broader struggle for human rights. Malcolm X said that the movement ought to be called a struggle for human rights instead of civil rights (Wronka, 2008). Martin Luther King Jr. argued that the civil rights movement had moved into a new era of human rights (quoted in Wronka, 2008).

Second generation rights correlate to the Eastern region of Soviet bloc communist countries that prioritized, at least in political theory, economic, social, and cultural rights such as the rights to health, work, adequate standard of living, social security, and social services. The second generation of human rights is a natural fit with social work. Mainstays of the profession, such as social security, maternal and infant care, and social services, are specifically mentioned. Social work priorities such as ensuring an adequate standard of living, health, education, and other social goals are enumerated. Third generation rights correlate with the non-aligned block, or the so-called third world (that is, in fact, the same "third" in the same sense), which prioritizes solidarity and collective rights such as the rights to peace, development, cultural and linguistic preservation, and environmental sustainability.

Many social work texts on human rights replicate this model (Ife, 2012; Reichert, 2011). However, despite its uses as a representational theoretical model for grasping the various components of human rights, it serves to reinforce the divisions and disagreements that led to the different generations. Despite being commonly associated with second generation rights, social work is very concerned with first generation rights, for example in its respect for diversity and attention to discrimination, and in its services to torture survivors and other victims of violations of civil and political rights. Social work has also always worked towards third generation rights, particularly in its advocacy for peace (Addams, 1922; Sanders &

Matsuoka, 1989) and in social development (Midgley, 2014). Furthermore, social work's emphasis upon holistic practice that attends to the "whole person" and situates people within their social environment via a human behavior in the social environment framework dissolves and looks beyond the generational divisions. Violations of civil and political rights have economic, social, and cultural consequences. The torture survivor and those who are denied free speech are likely to have negative health and mental health consequences. Conversely, violations of solidarity rights have civil and political consequences including a lack of peace and a lack of development. And the violation of the right to environment has health implications. "Social workers . . . accept the premise . . . that the full realization of civil and political rights is impossible without enjoyment of economic, social and cultural rights" (UN, 1994, p. 5).

Civil and political rights were considered "legal" rights to be implemented immediately; economic and social rights were considered "program" rights to be implemented progressively through a system of periodic reports. Second generation rights were held to be separate and of a different nature from first generation rights, which were thought to be immediate and absolute (Claude & Weston, 2006). In contrast, the second generation of rights was considered needing to be realized gradually and progressively. The remedies for each set of rights were assumed to be different. Where first generation rights were seen to be justiciable, second generation rights were seen to be less under the purview of courts and the rule of law, but, rather, programmatic and the purview of government administration and policies. This is why second generation rights were also assumed to be more political than legal. Second generation rights are assumed to be achieved through political reform, social policy, and programs. This has led to critiques of second generation rights as requiring costly welfare state obligations, as opposed to free or cheap first generation rights that rely on the non-interference of state actors. The distinction between first and second generation rights reflects different values of freedom or equality and different cultural orientations, such as the Western emphasis on individuality and liberalism or the Eastern emphasis on collectivism and socialism (Marks, 2005).

These conceptualizations of the distinctions between and divisions among human rights permeated the rights discourse for decades. This terminology reflects an outdated conception of human rights that is linked to Cold War Era disputes between political and economic systems, and their meaning becomes diminished upon scrutiny. A broad consensus of the aspirational and inspirational Universal Declaration of Human Rights as indivisible masked a disagreement that emerged to the forefront when discussing how to implement human rights. This disagreement resulting in the splitting of human rights between the two Covenants along generational lines. Consensus regarding the interdependence of rights reflected in the Universal Declaration was lost when the UN moved on to the conventions, which is why many of the rights included in the UDHR were "divided" between the two Covenants. As a human rights culture develops, all rights eventually become justiciable and codified by law in political systems. Finally, all rights require investment of resources.

This framework for practice integrates all three generations of human rights. Each of the five principles for practice applies equally to each set of rights in any of the generations. A common theme that animates all five of these principles is that of "humanization" or re-humanization. Recognizing and realizing each other's full humanity. Social work should be crucial to that, and rights-based approaches can accomplish this. Human rights are "a powerful discourse that seeks to overcome divisiveness and sectarianism and to unite people of different cultural and religious traditions in a single movement asserting human values and the universality of humanity" (Ife, 2012, p. 9). Dignity and nondiscrimination humanize people, nondiscrimination and participation ensure inclusiveness and belonging, and transparency and accountability incorporate justice into practice.

References

Addams, J. (1922). *Peace and bread in the time of war*. New York: Macmillan.

Albrithen, A., & Androff, D. (in press). The convergence of social work and human rights: Analyzing the historical and ethical foundations of allied disciplines. *Indian Journal of Social Work*.

Allan, J., Briskman, L., & Pease, B. (Eds.). (2009). *Critical social work: Theories and practices for a socially just world* (2nd ed.). Crows Nest, Australia: Allen & Unwin.

Androff, D. (2013). Human rights violations in the war on immigration. In A. Ackerman & R. Furman (Eds.), *Criminalization of immigration: Contexts and consequences*. Durham, NC: Carolina Academic Press.

Androff, D., & McPherson, J. (2014). Can human rights-based social work practice bridge the micro/macro divide? In K. Libal, M. Berthold, R. Thomas, & L. Healy (Eds.), *Advancing human rights in social work education* (pp. 23–40). Alexandria, VA: CSWE Press.

Baderin, M., & McCorquodale, R. (2007). *Economic, social, and cultural rights in action*. Oxford: Oxford University Press.

Berthold, M. (2015). Human rights-based approaches to clinical social work. In S. Gatenio Gabel (Ed.), *Springer briefs in rights-based approaches to social work series*. New York: Springer.

Burns, J. (2009). Mental health and inequity: A human rights approach to inequality, discrimination, and mental disability. *Health & Human Rights, 11*(2), 19–31.

Claude, R., & Weston, B. (Eds.). (2006). *Human rights in the world community: Issues and action* (3rd ed.). Philadelphia: University of Pennsylvania Press.

Cocker, C., & Hafford-Letchfield, T. (Eds.). (2014). *Rethinking anti-discriminatory and anti-oppressive theories for social work practice*. New York: Palgrave Macmillan.

Cornwall, A. (2008). Unpacking 'participation': models, meanings, and practices. *Community Development Journal, 43*(3), 269–283.

Council on Social Work Education (CSWE). (2008). *Educational Policy and Accreditation Standards*. Alexandria, VA: Author. Retrieved from: www.cswe.org/File.aspx?id=41861

Council on Social Work Education (CSWE). (2011). *Recovery to Practice: Developing Mental Health Recovery in Social Work*. Alexandria, VA: Author. Retrieved from: www.cswe.org/File.aspx?id=51135

Dalrymple, J., & Burke, B. (2006). *Anti-oppressive practice: Social care and the law* (2nd ed.). Buckingham: Open University.

Dominelli, L. (2002). *Anti-oppressive social work theory and practice*. New York: Palgrave Macmillan.

Dominelli, L. (2012). *Green social work: From environmental crises to environmental justice*. Cambridge: Polity.

Ezell, M. (2001). *Advocacy in the human services*. Belmont, CA: Wadsworth/Thomson.

Fook, J. (2012). *Social work: A critical approach to practice* (2nd ed.). Thousand Oaks, CA: Sage.

Freire, P. (2000). *Pedagogy of the oppressed*. New York: Continuum International.

Gatenio Gabel, S. (2015). Foreword, in K. Libal & S. Harding, Rights-based approaches to community practice (pp. v–xv). In S. Gatenio Gabel (Ed.), *Springer briefs in rights-based approaches to social work*. New York: Springer.

Gilbert, N., & Terrell, P. (2012). *Dimensions of social welfare policy* (8th ed.). New York: Pearson.

Hardiman, E., & Hodges, J. (2008). Professional differences in attitudes toward and utilization of psychiatric recovery. *Families in Society, 89*(2), 220–227.

Healy, L. (2008). *International social work: Professional action in an interdependent world* (2nd ed.). Oxford: Oxford University Press.

Huenchuan, S., & Rodriguez-Pinero, L. (2011). *Ageing and the protection of human rights: Current situation and outlook*. UN report. Santiago, Chile: Economic Commission for Latin America and the Caribbean. Retrieved from: http://social.un.org/ageing-working-group/documents/ECLAC_Ageing and the protection of human rights_current situation and outlook_Project document.pdf

Ife, J. (2012). *Human rights and social work: Towards rights-based practice* (3rd ed.). Cambridge: Cambridge University Press.

International Association of Schools of Social Work, International Federation of Social Workers, & International Council on Social Welfare (IASWW, IFSW & ICSW). (2012). *Global Agenda for Social Work and Social Development: Commitment to Action*. Retrieved from: www.globalsocialagenda.org/

Jones, A. (2005). The case of CARE International in Rwanda. In P. Gready & J. Ensor (Eds.), *Reinventing development: Translating rights-based approaches from theory into practice* (pp. 79–98). London: Zed Books.

Libal, K., & Harding, S. (2015). *Human rights-based community practice in the United States*. In S. Gatenio Gabel (Ed.), *Springer briefs in rights-based approaches to social work series*. New York: Springer.

Lundy, C. (2011). *Social work, social justice and human rights: A structural approach to practice* (2nd ed.). Toronto: University of Toronto Press.

Mandela, N. (2005). *Mandela's poverty speech*. BBC News. Retrieved from: http://news.bbc.co.uk/2/hi/uk_news/politics/4232603.stm

Marks, S. (2005). The human rights framework for development: Seven approaches. In A. Sengupta, A. Negi, & M. Basu (Eds.), *Reflections on the right to development* (pp. 23–60). New Delhi: Sage.

McPherson, J. (2012). Does narrative exposure therapy reduce PTSD in survivors of mass violence? *Research in Social Work Practice, 22*(1), 29–42.

McPherson, J. (2015). *Human rights practice in social work: A rights-based framework and two new measures* (Unpublished doctoral dissertation). Florida State University, Tallahassee.

Midgley, J. (2007). Development, social development, and human rights. In E. Reichert (Ed.), *Challenges in human rights* (pp. 97–121). New York: Columbia University Press.

Midgley, J. (2014). *Social development: Theory and practice*. Los Angeles: Sage.

Midgley, J., & Conley, A. (Eds.) (2010). *Social work and social development: Theories and skills for developmental social work*. Oxford: Oxford University Press.

Mullaly, R. (2007). *The new structural social work: Ideology, theory, practice* (3rd ed.). Oxford: Oxford University Press.

National Association of Social Workers (NASW). (2008). *Code of Ethics*. Washington, DC: Author. Retrieved from: www.socialworkers.org/pubs/code/code.asp

Nimmagadda, J., & Martell, D. (2008). Home-made social work: The two-way transfer of social work practice knowledge between India and the USA. In M. Gray, J. Coates, & M. Yellowbird (Eds.), *Indigenous social work around the world: Toward culturally relevant education and practice* (pp. 141–152). Burlington, VT: Ashgate.

Nipperess, S., & Briskman, L. (2009). Promoting a human rights perspective on critical social work. In J. Allan, L. Briskman, & B. Pease (Eds.), *Critical social work: Theories and practices for a socially just world* (2nd ed., pp. 58–69). Crows Nest, Australia: Allen & Unwin.

Nyamu-Musembi, C., & Cornwall, A. (2004). *What is the 'rights-based approach' all about? Perspectives from international development agencies.* IDS Working Paper 234. Brighton: Institute of Development Studies. Retrieved from: www.ids.ac.uk/files/dmfile/Wp234.pdf

Okitikpi, T., & Aymer, C. (2010). *Key concepts in anti-discriminatory social work.* Thousand Oaks, CA: Sage.

Pells, K. (2010). 'No one ever listens to us': Challenging obstacles to the participation of children and young people in Rwanda. In B. Percy-Smith & N. Thomas (Eds.), *A handbook of children and young people's participation: Perspectives from theory and practice* (pp. 196–203). Oxford: Routledge.

Reichert, E. (2011). *Social work and human rights: A foundation for policy and practice* (2nd ed.). New York: Columbia University Press.

Rothman, J., & Mizrahi, T. (2014). Balancing micro and macro practice: A challenge for social work. *Social Work, 59*(1), 91–93.

Sanders, D., & Matsuoka, J. (1989). *Peace and development: An interdisciplinary perspective.* Honolulu: University of Hawaii Press.

Thompson, N. (2012). *Anti-discriminatory practice: Equality, diversity and social justice* (5th ed.). Basingstoke: Palgrave Macmillan.

United Nations (UN). (1948, December 10). Universal Declaration of Human Rights. UN General Assembly. Retrieved from: www.un.org/Overview/rights.html

United Nations (UN). (1994). *Human Rights and Social Work. A Manual for Schools of Social Work and the Social Work Profession.* Professional Training Series No. 1. Geneva: Centre for Human Rights. Retrieved from: www.ohchr.org/documents/publications/training1en.pdf

United Nations (UN). (2001). *Seventeen frequently asked questions about United Nations Special Rapporteurs.* New York: Office of the High Commissioner for Human Rights. Retrieved from: www.ohchr.org/Documents/Publications/FactSheet27en.pdf

United Nations (UN). (2006). *Frequently asked questions on a human rights-based approach to development cooperation.* New York: Office of the United Nations High Commissioner for Human Rights. Retrieved from: www.ohchr.org/documents/publications/faqen.pdf

United Nations (UN). (2008). *Fact Sheet No. 31. The Right to Health.* New York: Office of the High Commissioner for Human Rights. Retrieved from: www.ohchr.org/Documents/Publications/Factsheet31.pdf

Wronka, J. (2008). *Human rights and social justice: Social action and service for the helping and health professions.* Thousand Oaks, CA: Sage.

Wronka, J., & Staub-Bernasconi, S. (2012). Human rights. In K. Lyons, T. Hokenstad, M. Pawar, N. Huegler, & N. Hall (Eds.), *The Sage handbook of international social work* (pp. 70–84). London: Sage.

3

HUMAN RIGHTS-BASED APPROACHES TO POVERTY

Traditional anti-poverty approaches in social work do not emphasize human rights. Given this, what do human rights mean to the poor? What is the value of human rights to the one fifth of humanity that lives without basic needs? While human rights are not commonly linked to poverty in Western countries such as the U.S., the poor and those in the Global South view the alleviation of poverty as a vital human rights struggle. Until it is overcome, poverty remains a fundamental challenge to human rights. It constitutes a grave and massive violation of one in five of all humans on earth; the magnitude and pervasiveness of poverty also threaten the basic value of human rights at all. A social work perspective demands the question: if human rights mean nothing to the least among us, then what are they worth? Human rights should be useful to the most vulnerable of populations – therefore this exploration of rights-based approaches begins by examining their applicability to those that social workers are professionally pledged to serve: the poor.

This section contains a brief introduction to the problem of poverty that the rest of the chapter will draw upon. It reviews common definitions, statistics, and traditional social work practice in the area of poverty to set context for identifying the human rights most pertinent to poverty.

Conceptions of poverty

Poverty is understood in different ways. Although to be poor is predominantly viewed as an economic status, the most common economic statistics such as gross domestic product do not indicate poverty rates; a nation's overall economic health does not capture poverty. Different conceptions and explanations of poverty are reflected in various measures of poverty. Poverty has been defined as a lack of income, deprivation, inequality, a lack of freedom, and oppression, and measured in absolute and relative terms.

Absolute measures of poverty understand the problem to be primarily economic and a lack of adequate income; an "absolute measure" is a level at which someone is considered to be poor or unable to meet their basic needs through their economic or material resources. The widely publicized UN figure of the people in the world living on less than one U.S. dollar a day is an absolute measure of poverty, as are most national poverty lines. In contrast, relative measures of poverty consider the number of people that are poor relative to others in the same country or society. Relative measures contextualize poverty and indicate inequality within societies. Defining poverty as a function of insufficient income is convenient for measurement and categorization purposes but fails to grasp the severity and reality of material deprivation. Recognizing this limitation, alternative measures of poverty have been developed to extend the concept beyond just economics.

Nobel Laureate Amartya Sen (1999) reconceptualized poverty as a lack of freedom that constricts people's choices to live a life that they value, undertake meaningful action, and pursue self-directed goals. Sen recognized that poverty constrains people's ability to take action, and proposed that development, insofar as an anti-poverty initiative, should result in greater freedom for its beneficiaries. Philosopher Martha Nussbaum (2011) has furthered this into the "capabilities approach", drawing upon the concept of human capital in acknowledging that it is people's capacity for self-directed goal fulfillment, to make choices and take action, which contributes to their well-being.

The Human Development Index is another measure that conceives of poverty in terms of human well-being rather than economics, as a limit to the extent of human development that people and a society can achieve. This measure is well publicized in the UN Development Program's annual Human Development Report (2014). A major strength of the Human Development Index is its simplicity; it combines five social indicators of life expectancy, education levels, and income (gross national income per capita). The UN Committee on Economic, Social and Cultural Rights combines many of these approaches in its multi-dimensional understanding of poverty as chronic deprivation of an adequate standard of living due to lack of resources, capabilities, choices, security, and power (Marks, 2013). The multidimensional poverty index incorporates interconnected dimensions of deprivations of health, education, and standards of living. It is based on the intensity of poverty and calculates the average number of deprivations experienced by each household and the number of people per household in "multidimensional poverty".

Social exclusion is a conception of poverty that refers less to material deprivation, lack of income, lack of human capital, or personal failure, but to the lack of participation in and building up of community, and access to social capital (Wronka, 2008). All these measures are important in understanding the link between human rights, social work, and poverty. As will be developed further in this chapter, rights-based approaches typically extend this view of poverty as the result of a lack of participation in all aspects of social life.

Extent of poverty

Global estimates

Absolute measures of poverty depend entirely on the decision of where to set the dollar amount (using U.S. dollars for our purposes here). For example, if we raise the typical demarcations of $1.00, $1.25, or $2.50 to $10.00, then our sense of poverty changes dramatically (especially from a Western, relatively rich perspective). 80% of the world's population lives on less than $10 a day. Half of the world's population lives on less than $2.50 (UNDP, 2014).

The World Bank measures global poverty using the absolute measure of a poverty line at $1.25 per day in 2005 prices, which is the mean of 15 of the poorest countries' national poverty lines (World Bank, 2013). Based on this research, the World Bank estimates that in 2008 about 1.28 billion people lived below this line (World Bank, 2013). This is 20.63%, or 1 in 5 people. This figure is down from 1.9 billion in 1990 (World Bank, 2013). In 2010, this was estimated to be 726.75 million people, or 12.34% of the world's population (World Bank, 2013).

The poverty line of $2.00 a day is also commonly used, and speaks more to middle-income countries. In fact, it is the mean of the national poverty lines of these countries (World Bank, 2013). The number of the poor, measured as those living on less than $2 a day, has declined from 2.59 billion in 1981 to 2.4 billion in 2010 (Marks, 2013). Considering the world's population growth during that time, this represents a decrease of over 20% in the world's population.

Using the multidimensional poverty index, an estimated 1.56 billion people live in poverty. This number is greater than the 1.14 billion living on less than $1.25 per day – but less than the number surviving on less than $2.00 per day (UNDP, 2014).

Regional estimates

There are many regional differences in the global distribution of poverty. Using the same data as above (World Bank, 2013), South Asia is the region with the highest number of people in poverty, 506.77 million, or 31.03% of the population. Sub-Saharan Africa is the region with the highest percentage of people in poverty, at 48.47%, or 413.73 million people. The East Asia and Pacific region have the next highest number of people in poverty, at 250.9 million, and percentage of the population in poverty, at 12.48%. The region including Latin America and the Caribbean has the next highest poverty rate, 32.20 million people, or 5.53%. The least amount of data is available for the region of the Middle East and North Africa, although it is reported that there are 7.98 million people in poverty, or 2.41% of the population. Eastern Europe and Central Asia have lower rates of poverty, 3.15 million people or 0.66% of the population.

Using the $2.00 per day poverty line, from 1981 to 2005 the percent of the population of Sub-Saharan Africa only decreased slightly from 74% to 73%, although the actual number of persons under the $2 line grew from 294 million to 557 million. Highlighting stark regional contrasts, in East Asia the number of people living on less than $2 a day fell from 1.28 billion in 1981, or 95.4% of the region's population, to 0.73 billion in 2005, or 38.7% (Marks, 2013).

Poverty outliers

The UNDP and World Bank classify countries into four categories: low income, low-middle income, high-middle income, and high income. Based on the multi-dimensional poverty index (MPI), the four countries with the greatest percentage of people in poverty are all in Africa, and include Ethiopia (87%), Liberia (84%), Mozambique (79%), and Sierra Leone (77%). Although countries in the Global North have some of the lowest poverty rates, poverty does exist in countries with high overall human development. In many societies, poverty is a persistent presence – especially among vulnerable populations such as the homeless and ethnic minorities in urban centers and rural areas. Rights-based approaches to alleviating poverty are also relevant to pockets of poverty in the Global North.

Trends in declining global poverty and growing inequality

The last several years have seen dramatic reductions in global poverty. This includes the successful achievement of the first Millennium Development Goal, halving the world's population living on less than $1.25 a day by 2012, 3 years prior to the 2015 target. However, this anti-poverty progress is mainly due to significant advances in "super growth" economie of emerging countries, BRIC nations (Brazil, Russia, India, China). For example Brazil saw reduced the percentage of people living on less than $1.25 per day from 17.2% to 6.1%, and India from 49.4% to 32.7%. Over half of the world's progress in combating poverty occurred in China – which reduced the same population from 60.2% to 13.1%. China has been credited with lifting 510 million people from poverty (UNDP, 2014). In fact, the World Bank (2013) reports that most poverty reduction has occurred in China. Beyond China little progress has been seen, and in some regions such as Sub-Saharan Africa, poverty has worsened. This case, Sub-Saharan Africa, is an important regional caveat to be considered. Around the world there is a widening gap between the wealthiest and the poorest members of the same countries and regions (UNDP, 2014). The 2008 global financial crisis stalled economic development and set back poverty reduction. Many states have continued to struggle to find austerity, stimulus, or a combination of policies to promote economic growth.

Why start with poverty?

This book explores a number of social problems, so why does it begin with poverty? This choice is due to the centrality of the problem of poverty to the people of the world and to social work. Poverty is recognized as a massive social problem and threat to global well-being, and is one of the chief problems that social workers confront. This is reflected in the first Millennium Development Goal, eradicating extreme poverty between 1990 and 2015 (Mapp, 2014). Poverty is complex, multi-dimensional, and connected to many social ills; poverty is the social problem that makes all the others worse and often a common denominator to other problems. Children are especially vulnerable to poverty and suffer the worst consequences of living in poverty; in the U.S. one in five children live in poverty – the age-group with the highest rate of poverty. Older adults are the most vulnerable to becoming poor; historically, and still in many parts of the world, to grow old was to risk becoming poor. Health problems are also compounded by poverty: the poor face greater health risks, suffer more health problems, and health costs often contribute to poverty. In the U.S., health care costs are the leading cause of bankruptcy. Poverty has been shown to cause stress and exacerbate psychosocial distress. Consequently people suffering from mental health or developmental disabilities are at a high risk for poverty. Poverty has been conceptualized as a form of violence called structural violence – because when poverty is a part of a socially unjust social system, it is causing harm to those that suffer from it. The structural dimensions of poverty include unequal access to resources, unequal participation in the marketplace, and unjust governance. Therefore poverty affects many dimensions of professional social work practice.

There is a growing recognition of the link between human rights and poverty. In 2006, for the first time, the Nobel Peace Prize was awarded in recognition of anti-poverty work to the Grameen Bank and its founder Muhammad Yunus. This decision recognized the important link between poverty and peace, violence, and social stability. Human rights organizations such as Amnesty International and Human Rights Watch have conducted investigations and issued reports on poverty as a violation of economic human rights. Rights-based approaches to economic development are becoming mainstream in the UN and among major development organizations; rights-based approaches to practice among non-governmental organizations are emerging (Jones, 2005). Policymakers increasingly perceive human rights as instrumental for poverty reduction (Marks, 2013).

Poverty is also a topic where the strongest connections are found between human rights and social work. Poverty is a natural starting place due to the historical commitment of the social work profession. Indeed, poverty remains a part of the central focus of the social work profession around the world. In this gambit to transform social work practice, it is necessary to start in the heart of the profession to reanimate its core social justice function.

Traditional approaches to poverty

Poverty has long been a central focus of the social work profession. Some have argued that poverty remains the defining feature of the social work profession, distinguishing social work professional practice from psychology or medicine. However, others have argued that social workers have not preserved this historical commitment and instead have pursued more lucrative and less pressing concerns (Specht & Courtney, 1994).

Social work approaches to poverty have historically been influenced by social policies rooted in the model of the Elizabethan Poor Laws and the Progressive Era's settlement movement and Charity Organization Societies, which viewed poverty as a moral deficiency (Abramovitz, 1988). Interventions were characterized by paternalism, featuring reactive, emergency, short-term assistance that provided only a minimum amount of aid. Policies and programs were framed as charity, based on a residual approach that prioritizes the responsibility of families, faith-based organizations, and communities, and emphasized residency requirements to receive aid. "Friendly visitors", forerunners to professionals, spent time with poor families to encourage them to overcome their personal failings.

In contrast, the settlement movement's understanding of poverty included multiple factors such as environmental stressors, lack of English language and other skills, poor working conditions, and low pay. Their approach to poverty was characterized by environmental and neighborhood change, increasing people's human capital, and fostering social integration and civic participation. While the settlement movement was influential among many reform movements in the late 19th and early 20th centuries, it is the Charity Organization Society's approach that has colored many contemporary approaches.

Global poverty was taken as a sign of the inferiority of nations and cultures to the colonizers from the West. In the 20th century, global poverty was understood to be a precondition to free market capitalist development. U.S. President Harry Truman in 1945 coined the term "underdeveloped countries" to underscore the idea of a singular progressive path of development based on modernization and industrialization theories of economic growth. The concept of development, similar to how the concept of poverty has been refined and broadened, has been expanded to human development, meaning the improvement of the well-being, quality of life, and greater freedom for a community.

Many contemporary anti-poverty programs function as income subsidies, and provide poor beneficiaries cash payments on the basis of categorical programs (Midgley, 2010). Rooted in a charity approach, contemporary approaches to poverty remain mainly residual, reflecting primarily an economic deficiency view of poverty. In many anti-poverty programs, eligibility is determined by means-testing and is characterized by meager, temporary benefits, minimum subsistence to the most desperate of the poor. These programs have been found to have a coercive, social control function, particularly of women and minorities (Abramovitz, 1988).

Social work roles include the case worker or case management approach – where professionals help their clients to navigate bureaucratic structures, complicated policies, applications, and restrictions. This approach has a distinctly micro-focus, with the practitioner focusing on remedying or attending to the individual's most pressing needs. Social workers may act as a broker of supportive and remedial services, such as counseling or services to assist with other personal problems that the individual is experiencing.

Social policies and programs designed to address poverty (typically in the U.S. and the West) have been politically attacked and criticized for enabling a "welfare dependency" with perverse incentives that discourage people from taking corrective action to exit poverty, such as hard work, self-denial, and discipline. Such critiques, along with highly publicized cases of welfare fraud, contributed to crises of public confidence in many welfare states, leading to policy reforms including punitive eligibility and enforcement measures.

Recently, alternative approaches have gathered attention such as social development which emphasizes integrating social and economic policies through social investments in people's capabilities, and human and social capital (Midgley, 2014). Asset based development, including micro-credit and micro-enterprise programs, have gained popularity in social work circles (Lindsey, 2003; Sherraden & Stevens, 2010). Internationally, social work is involved in asset development work in Sub-Saharan Africa (Ssewamala, Sperber, Zimmerman & Karimli, 2010), developmental social work in South Africa (Midgley & Conley, 2010), and conditional cash transfers in Mexico, Brazil, and Indonesia (Gatenio Gabel & Kamerman, 2008).

The human right to be free from poverty

Central to rights-based approaches to poverty is the idea that every human being has the right to a life that is free from poverty. There is now a widespread consensus that poverty violates human rights (Despouy, 1996; Pogge, 2011). The Vienna Declaration, from the 1993 World Conference on Human Rights, affirmed that extreme poverty inhibits human rights (UN, 1993). The World Health Organization called extreme poverty the world's greatest killer and source of suffering (WHO, 1995). The UN Commissioner for Human Rights identified extreme poverty as the most serious violation of human rights (UNDP, 2003). The former UN Secretary-General, Kofi Annan, said that "wherever we lift one soul from a life of poverty, we are defending human rights. And whenever we fail in this mission, we are failing human rights" (Annan, 2001, p. x).

This section identifies which human rights apply to poverty through a review of the core human rights documents that address poverty. The human right to be free from poverty is contained in the 1948 Universal Declaration of Human Rights, International Covenant on Economic, Social, and Cultural Rights (ICESCR), the Declaration on the Right to Development, and the Millennium Development Goals. Additionally there are human rights institutions that relate to poverty such as the Economic and Social Council, UN Development Program (UNDP), and the Committee on Economic, Social, and Cultural Rights which interprets relevant human rights instruments and monitors the ICESCR.

What do social workers need to know about human rights and poverty?

The human right to be free from poverty, along with other human rights related to basic human needs or survival rights – which are defined as essential for sustaining human life – have often been termed economic, social, and cultural rights. They are also known as second generation rights and often conceptualized as rights to social goods, such as a human's right to adequate nutrition, education, and others. As such, they are considered positive rights, as in the right "to" something actual and positive, in contrast to negative rights, such as the right to be free from torture or interference from the state. Social work scholars, as well as many in the human rights community, have problematized this distinction (Claude & Weston, 2006; Ife, 2012; Staub-Bernasconi, 2007). These terms reflect different conceptualizations of human rights and disagreement on the best way to achieve or implement rights, controversies about the prioritization of different types of rights, and historical disputes regarding competing economic and political systems.

For example, one could frame economic rights as negative rights, as in someone's right to be free from poverty. One could also conceive of the right to be free from poverty as the right to be free from state influence, in the form of exploitative policies and practices, international labor and trade agreements, and from multi-national corporations. In fact, this book uses the phrase "the human right to be free from poverty" instead of "the human right to an adequate standard of living" or "the human right to development". Similarly, what is the point of saving someone from torture only for them to die in a famine? What is the use of distinguishing between first and second generation of rights when for example government repression is the cause of violations of both torture and famine, with the same consequences in human costs? This division misses the indivisible and interconnected reality of human rights; the intersectionality of rights recognizes that splitting or prioritizing rights leads to false dichotomies and misunderstandings of how rights are enjoyed or violated.

The history of economic rights rhetoric in the U.S. reveals the interconnected roots between first and second generations of rights. Franklin D. Roosevelt's 1941 State of the Union address included the freedom from want in his list of four essential human freedoms, along with the freedom of speech, the freedom of worship, and the freedom from fear. President Roosevelt identified personal economic security as fundamental to peace and stability among nations. The freedom from want refers to a conceptualization of poverty as deprivation. Roosevelt also called for an Economic Bill of Rights, in response to the national recognition that individual liberty is dependent upon economic security and independence. However, this early linkage or common identification of economic rights was overshadowed by the post-World War II political divide in which the democracies of the West were contrasted with the Eastern socialist and communist states. This geopolitical divide resulted in the U.S. opposing economic rights, despite Roosevelt's initial support, fracturing the human rights community and discourse for decades. Human rights proponents spoke past each other, with the West criticizing communist states' lack of civil and political freedoms and communist countries criticizing the West's lack of social and economic rights.

One result of this division in terms of poverty is that economic and social rights are neglected and treated as less of a priority than civil and political rights. The historical dimensions of how the debate has evolved influenced the development of human rights approaches (Staub-Bernasconi, 2007). This furthered the exclusion of the poor and engendered resistance to human rights for the poor, such as the right to development (Sengupta, 2006). Fortunately the current trend now is towards holistic views of human rights, the inclusion of the poor in human rights, and rights-based approaches to development. Presently it is generally accepted, as Roosevelt outlined over 70 years ago, that freedom and equality are co-requisites.

Universal Declaration of Human Rights (UDHR)

Poverty is a violation of human rights, both of specific rights, such as the right to an adequate standard of living, but also of the spirit of human rights exemplified by the principle of human dignity. Article 25 of the Universal Declaration of Human Rights (UN, 1948) provides for the human right to be free from poverty: "Everyone has the right to a standard of living adequate for the health and well-being of himself and of his family, including food, clothing, housing, and medical care and necessary social services, and the right to security in the event of unemployment, sickness, disability, widowhood, old age or other lack of livelihood in circumstances beyond his control. Motherhood and childhood are entitled to special care and assistance. All children, whether born in or out of wedlock, shall enjoy the same social protection".

The right to work is commonly how the human right to an adequate standard of living is conceptualized. The path of work, employment, and livelihood has long been recognized as central to many of life's essential objectives (Nickel, 2007). The international community's commitment to the right to work and its recognition of the role of work in the welfare of people's lives can be traced at least to the International Labour Organization's (ILO) founding in 1919. During the drafting of the UDHR, the ILO advocated linking the right to social goods such as food and health to an adequate standard of living. Provided that people can freely choose their work, earn sufficient income, and labor under safe conditions, the right to work has profound anti-poverty implications. For example, fair and accessible opportunities to earn living wages can lead to poverty reduction through the workplace and market-based exchanges.

International Covenant on Economic, Social and Cultural Rights (ICESCR)

The International Covenant on Economic, Social and Cultural Rights (ICESCR), established in 1966 and entered into force in 1976, is currently ratified by 162 nations (UN, 1966). U.S. President Jimmy Carter signed it in 1978, but Congress never ratified it as required by the U.S. Constitution. The ICESCR focuses on a range of economic, social, and cultural rights in the areas of employment, social security, education, health care, and participation in cultural and scientific activities. The ICESCR is among the foremost documents addressing the right to be free from poverty.

The initial articles of the ICESCR assert everyone's right to self-determination to freely pursue their own economic, social, and cultural development (Reichert, 2011). People's economic well-being is recognized as important, regardless of their nation's political or economic system. States are expected to contribute to the realization of people's economic rights through the development and implementation of national laws and policies. The ICESCR makes exceptions for states during economic crises (Reichert, 2011), acknowledging that the realization of economic rights depends upon the availability of necessary resources and must be implemented progressively (Midgley, 2007).

Core rights in the ICESCR relevant to poverty are the rights to work and to social security. Features of the right to work include the right to freely choose one's employment, the right to just and favorable working conditions, and the right to unionize. Article 6 specifies the human right to a livelihood through work, and that states are responsible for providing technical and vocational training and policies and programs that enable people to achieve their economic development. This responsibility is necessary for people to achieve full and productive employment, and to maintain individual economic liberty. Article 7 highlights the rights to just and favorable work conditions, which include fair and equal remuneration, safe and healthy working conditions, equal opportunity for promotion, and rest, leisure, and reasonable limitation of working hours and periodic holidays. Article 8 guarantees the right to form and join trade unions, including the right to strike; exceptions are presented in cases of national security and public order. Article 9 contains the right to social security and social insurance. Article 10 sets out rights related to the family unit, including the right of spouses to freely consent to enter into marriage, protects the human right to compensated maternity leave, and children from economic exploitation. Article 11 recognizes the right to an adequate standard of living, which includes the right to food, clothing, housing, and the continuous improvement of living conditions. This article also notes that international cooperation is required for multi-state issues such as food production and distribution.

The right to development

Economic development through market-based growth remains the main anti-poverty mechanism for most states and global institutions. However economic development does not equal human development and it has become clear that economic growth is insufficient. The limits of markets, such as global recessions, crises, and distorted development mean that economic growth may not benefit everyone, and can result in greater inequality (Midgely, 2007).

Human rights have been predominantly linked to political rather than economic goals, such as democratization and strengthening the rule of law. Market-based solutions to poverty reduction raise the question of whether development, as the process of economic growth, can be considered a human right. Connections between human rights and economic development include a focus on participation and social development, and have fostered a rights-based turn in development (Marks, 2013).

History

The right to development movement originated from the non-aligned movement of nations recovering from decolonization and resisting the dominant world powers' political struggles in the UN and international affairs (Midgley, 2007). The first call for a right to development was made by Judge Keba M'Baye of Senegal in a 1972 lecture at the International Institute of Human Rights. The idea gained acceptance as the international community struggled to deal with the consequences of globalization, including increased international debt, global poverty, and environmental degradation (Midgley, 2007).

The right to development was codified in the 1986 Declaration on the Right to Development and reaffirmed in 1993 at the second UN World Conference on Human Rights and its resulting Vienna Declaration (Sengupta, 2006). This consensus began to resolve the Cold War dichotomization of mutually exclusive first and second generation rights and led to the 1995 UN World Summit on Social Development and the resulting Copenhagen Declaration. The 2000 Millennium Development Goals invoked the right to development and its connection to freedom from want (UN, 2013). These statements explicitly emphasized the link between development and human rights, and recognized the need for peace, security, and fundamental freedoms as a necessary condition for development and social justice (Midgley, 2007).

Definition

The right to development is based upon the UDHR's Article 28, which stipulates the right to a stable international social order, and the ICESCR's Article 1, which asserts the right to self-determination for human development (Midgley, 2007). Article 1 of the 1986 Declaration of the Right to Development defines this right as the right "to participate in, contribute to, and enjoy" development (UN, 1986). The Declaration defines development as "a comprehensive economic, social, cultural, and political process" for the purpose of "the constant improvement of the well-being of the entire population and of all individuals, on the basis of their active, free and meaningful participation in development and in the fair distribution of benefits resulting therefrom" (UN, 1986). The Working Group on the Right to Development 2010 called the right to development "the right of peoples and individuals to the constant improvement of their well-being and to a national and global enabling environment conducive to just, equitable, participatory, and human-centered development respectful of all human rights" (quoted in Marks, 2013, p. 23). The right to development conceives of participation to mean active, free, and meaningful, and of equitable to mean the fair distribution of benefits.

The right to development contributes to the elimination of poverty through its attention to goals of comprehensive and human-centered development policy, participatory processes, and to distributing the benefits and burdens of development in a socially just manner. The right to development extends an economic definition of poverty towards social and human development conceptualizations that acknowledge that human dignity and respect should be inherent in development processes. In addition to meeting basic needs and building assets and wealth, development should contribute to people's well-being by maximizing human choices, expanding their freedom to achieve whatever they value in life (Sen, 1999), and increasing people's capacity to lead a life that they value (Nussbaum, 2011). The right to development aims to put people at the center of development and emphasizes the right of everyone to participate in development, particularly the vulnerable that may traditionally lose out on development projects. Collectively, people should be the primary subject, participant, and beneficiary of development. The right to development is distinct from other economic rights, as a right to a process rather than a standard. The right to participate in the process of development includes equality of opportunity, access to resources, and fair distribution of benefits. In order to be considered rights-based, the process of development must be open for all to participate; distorted development or development that compromises other human rights cannot be rights-based. The right to development would mean that a population in poverty and deprivation experiences rising standards of living and increased capacity to improve their position, leading to an increase in overall well-being for everyone.

Duties and obligations

States bear primary responsibility for implementing the human right to development; individuals are the beneficiaries (Sengupta, 2001). Article 2(2) of the Declaration of the Right to Development states that "All human beings, individually and collectively, have a responsibility for securing the right to development", but primary responsibility rests upon the state, and international cooperation is heavily emphasized (UN, 1986). The right to development is recognized as a duty of the state to set policies ensuring "equality of opportunity for all in their access to basic resources, education, health services, food, housing, employment, and the fair distribution of income" as well as participatory and equitable development policies. States are responsible for favorable development conditions and for eliminating obstacles to development. The Declaration calls for international cooperation when states are unable to create these conditions or remove obstacles on their own, with the goal of an international economic order that rests on sovereignty, equality, and interdependence.

States in the Global South have used the right to development to raise concerns about protectionist trade policies, disparities in technological access, and high levels of debt burdens and to argue that rich states have obligations to facilitate rights-based development. States in the Global North have used the right to development to argue for reforms encouraging good governance, anti-corruption, and rule of law (Marks, 2013).

Millennium Development Goals (MDGs)

The Millennium Development Goals (MDGs) comprise eight interrelated goals with over 40 measurable indicators, to be met by 2015, as measured from social indicators from 1990, based on the 1995 Copenhagen Summit on Social Development and subsequent 2000 Millennium Declaration, signed by 189 nations (Mapp, 2014). The first goal is to halve the number of people in the world living on less than $1.25 (USD) per day and to reduce the number of people in hunger by one half. The World Bank declared that the first goal has been met, reporting a decline of 52.2%, from 43.1% in 1990 to 20.6% (Marks, 2013). Unfortunately an estimated 1 billion people remain in extreme poverty (less than $1.25/day) and while there has been progress on reducing the number of people in hunger, the second part of the first goal has yet to be met. The MDGs have been criticized for failing to sufficiently integrate human rights (Marks, 2013); however, some links between the Millennium Development Goals and human rights have been made (UN, 2008; UNDP, 2007). Post-2015 planning efforts have included a greater human rights focus (Marks, 2013). Rights-based approaches should be included in the Sustainable Development Goals; this would ensure that the developmental agenda regards poverty as a violation of human rights.

Additional human rights mechanisms relating to poverty

In 1990 the UN Commission on Human Rights appointed a Special Rapporteur on Extreme Poverty and Human Rights, Arjun Sengupta, who published reports and academic papers on the right to development and later founded the Center for Development and Human Rights (Marks, 2013; Wronka, 2008). In 1998 the UN created an Independent Expert on Human Rights and Extreme Poverty and dialogue continued between UN agencies on developing human rights-based approaches to poverty reduction (UN, 2004). The Special Rapporteur on Extreme Poverty and Human Rights' guiding principles for policymakers on poverty reduction were adopted by the UN Human Rights Council in 2012. This was followed by an Advisory Committee's report on strategies and best practices for rights-based approaches for the urban poor. The Special Rapporteur continues to issue country reports, solicit contributions from NGOs, and highlight special issues, such as access to water and sanitation.

In 1998 the UN Commission on Human Rights established the Intergovernmental Working Group on the Right to Development which monitors progress towards the Declaration of the Right to Development and makes recommendations for programs and technical assistance for interested countries for implementation. The UN uses two commemorative days to raise global awareness on human rights and poverty. October 17 is the International Day for the Eradication of Extreme Poverty, created by Joseph Wresinski, the founder of the International Fourth World Movement to promote a just social order in which everyone enjoys human rights and dignity (Wronka, 2008). December 4 is the Right to Development Day, which commemorates the 1986 endorsement of the Declaration on the Right to Development and calls for structural economic and social reforms to promote equality of opportunity and elimination of social injustice (Wronka, 2008).

This chapter has focused on international frameworks that link human rights and poverty. However, at the regional level there are several human rights charters, agreements, and documents that promote economic rights. These include the European Social Charter (which is not required for new members to the Council of Europe to ratify, unlike the European Convention on Human Rights), the Additional Protocol of the American Convention on Human Rights, the African Charter on Human and People's Rights, and the Protocol of San Salvador. This last was an additional protocol adopted in 1988 by the Organization of American States. This does include economic rights but was only approved by 11 out of 25 members.

Case study of a rights-based approach to poverty

This section presents rights-based approaches to poverty alleviation and development. This chapter's primary case is drawn from the U.S. The book as a whole endeavors to use case examples from around the world to illustrate the global relevance of rights-based approaches. However, it is important to begin by acknowledging the persistent reality of human rights violations and the need to work for economic rights in the U.S. Social workers may appreciate the need for a necessary corrective to American human rights rhetoric, which is often perceived as hypocritical. Other cases are presented after the main case study before the following section on implications for social work practice.

Poor people's economic human rights campaign – United States

One case example of a rights-based approach to poverty in the U.S. is the Poor People's Economic Human Rights Campaign (PPEHRC) (Jewell, Collins, Gargotto & Dishon, 2009; Reichert, 2011; Wronka, 2008). The PPEHRC is a national non-governmental organization led by poor and homeless Americans raising the issue of poverty as a human rights violation. PPEHRC works with a coalition of community-based organizations and advocacy groups who promote social justice and human rights, including Arise for Social Justice (Springfield, MA), Kensington Welfare Rights Union (Philadelphia, PA), Social Welfare Action Alliance (national), among others (Wronka, 2008). The PPEHRC aims to end poverty through advancing economic human rights by uniting the poor across racial lines into a broad social movement (www.ppehrc.org).

Established in 1998, the PPEHRC was motivated by the failure to reduce poverty of the 1996 welfare reform policy Temporary Assistance to Needy Families (TANF). The PPEHRC argued that the U.S. violated economic rights with the TANF policy. The PPEHRC built upon the civil rights, welfare rights, and labor movements, and was created by members of the Kensington Welfare Rights Union in Philadelphia which has worked for economic human rights against poverty since 1991.

The PPEHRC has conducted many protests, marches, bus tours, regional and national summits, and staged demonstrations such as tent cities. They coordinated with the Pennsylvania chapter of the National Association of Social Workers, state legislators, and social work students to organize social workers in a successful push for a state level human rights legislative review.

In the process of encouraging and supporting poor people's participation, the PPEHRC has gathered documentation of economic human rights abuses and disseminated people's stories that had been affected by welfare reform in education campaigns, rallies, and public forums. In 2006 the PPEHRC held a Truth Commission to publicize poverty as a human rights violation. The Truth Commission consisted of testimonials documenting violations of the rights to health care, adequate standards of living, housing, water and sanitation, and education. Participants included more than 500 people living in poverty, human rights leaders, and artists and musicians who performed.

The PPEHRC have actively engaged with human rights mechanisms at the regional and international levels. Their advocacy has included testifying at the 2005 UN Regional Consultation on Women and the Right to Adequate Housing in North America before the UN Special Rapporteur on Adequate Housing and the Inter-American Commission on Human Rights. In 2013 the PPEHRC testified before the World Court for Women on economic human rights violations of women and children by global financial institutions.

The PPEHRC demonstrates the principles for rights-based practice of dignity, nondiscrimination, participation, transparency, and accountability. The PPEHRC focuses on human dignity by addressing the welfare of those left behind by the market economy and by society, who do not have the opportunity or access to enjoy an adequate standard of living. The dignity of the poor is respected because they are viewed as equal members of society, equal to all other members of the organization, professionals, officials, and leaders. The poor are not treated as deficient, maladapted, or in need of charitable pity; rather they are seen as people deserving of the same rights to an adequate standard of living, decent work, and freedom from poverty as everyone else. The PPEHRC's emphasis on building unity between people of different races, ethnicities, and classes into an inclusive social movement exemplifies the principle of nondiscrimination. The PPEHRC incorporated the principle of participation by design of having the leadership and membership of the organization comprised of poor people. The strategic interventions and tools used by the PPEHRC further embodied participation, specifically in their use of a Truth Commission.

Truth and Reconciliation Commissions (TRCs), as they are commonly referred to internationally, are community based, restorative justice models of promoting social change (Androff, 2010a) and have been used in the U.S. to address racial violence (Androff, 2010b; 2012a) and racial discrimination in housing and child welfare (Androff, 2012b). The participation of people who have suffered human rights violations through telling their stories at a TRC's public hearing provides individuals with support and validation (Androff, 2012c). The raising of people's voices who are typically excluded from public dialogue serves to raise awareness and promote transparency. By framing poverty as a human rights violation, the PPEHRC is cultivating political consciousness (Lakoff, 2004; Wronka, 2008). Raising awareness about the rights violations endured by the poor and educating people about their rights also increases transparency. The PPEHRC's use of a TRC also promotes accountability. The PPEHRC's advocacy at state, federal, regional, and international levels promotes the rights-based principle of accountability. Orchestrating and implementing a TRC requires many advocacy practice skills and interventions, such as community organizing (Androff, in press). The PPEHRC advocates for living wages and other social policies that respect the human right to be free from poverty. The advocacy of the PPEHRC is geared towards building a social movement that can hold governmental and financial actors accountable for economic human rights.

There are other examples of NGOs that are applying rights-based approaches to poverty. Oxfam International has adopted a rights-based approach to poverty that includes focus on the right to a sustainable livelihood, the right to basic social services, the right to life and security, the right to be heard in social and political arenas, and the right to an identity (Offenheiser & Holcombe, 2003; Sengupta, Negi & Basu, 2006). Oxfam defines poverty as a state of powerlessness that prohibits people from exercising their rights or control over their lives. Their rights-based approach puts the rights and interests of the poor at the center of their development and aid agenda.

Rights-based approaches to social work practice with poverty

Rights-based approaches to social work practice with poverty should encompass the principles of dignity, nondiscrimination, participation, transparency, and accountability. Human dignity, in terms of the human right to be free from poverty, means that practitioners should approach people living in poverty, not as needy objects of charity, but as rights-holders, deserving of fundamental human rights to be free from poverty, to benefit from development, and to have an adequate standard of living. Dignity emphasizes the social work value of self-determination. In a rights-based perspective, anti-poverty and development policies and programs are not discretionary, philanthropic, or altruistic but rather an entitlement based on international standards. The rights-based approach to development strengthens social development by moving beyond a needs-based approach and lending a specific framework, concrete and defined goals, and mechanisms (Midgley, 2007).

Nondiscrimination, in rights-based approaches to poverty, means that the poor have the right to be included in every aspect of society. Rights-based approaches promote social inclusion and inclusion in development activity, the market, and the workplace. A rights-based approach to poverty and development entails attending to the populations most affected by poverty and human rights violations. Nondiscrimination in a rights-based approach to practice with people in poverty means that social workers should recognize and attend to the intersectionality of oppression that blends discrimination, poverty, and myriad other conditions that violate rights and diminish well-being. In addition to the economic dimension of rights to be free from poverty, social workers should work to realize all the human rights of the poor; human rights are not a luxury of the wealthy but must be extended to the poor (Marks, 2013). Nondiscrimination also requires practitioners to bridge gaps of social class and other economic, social, and cultural divisions through personal reflection on bias and positionality in order to achieve non-hierarchical relationships.

Rights-based approaches also use participation to achieve social and economic transformation by and for the poor (Marks, 2013). Participation in rights-based approaches can include critical and transformative education that empowers poor people to take charge of their own lives and to have a voice in decisions and processes that affect their well-being. The principle of participation in social work practice includes asset, capacity, and community building to create and extend the abilities of the poor to influence, control, and hold accountable the institutions that affect their lives. Social workers should advocate for the right to join in trade unions which can have significant anti-poverty effects through the right to work, to fair and just working conditions, and to an adequate standard of living (Wronka, 2008).

Social workers can practice the principle of transparency through raising awareness of poor rights-holders through education about human rights and mobilization for action on anti-poverty campaigns (Marks, 2013). Transparency translates into social work practice in the area of assessment, which in rights-based approaches includes assessment of what human rights are being violated in addition to the right to be free from poverty. For people in poverty, there may be violations of the rights to housing, education, or health. Rights-based transparency in social work assessment examines specific violations' causation, which asks why someone is living in poverty; role, asking who bears responsibility for the right to be free from poverty; and capacity, analyzing what strengths, resources, and capabilities are required to overcome poverty. Transparency encompasses anti-corruption efforts in government, humanitarian aid and relief efforts, and elimination of waste and unnecessary overhead in social work practice, programs, and policies.

Accountability in rights-based approaches to poverty means that social workers should engage in advocacy (Marks, 2013). Rights-based approaches require greater emphasis on advocacy among service-delivery oriented practitioners (Kindornay, Ron & Carpenter, 2012). Social workers can use human rights to hold the powerful accountable to the weak. The material and financial resources required to end poverty and associated rights violations such as hunger and homelessness exist, but should be better leveraged to empower people to become free from poverty and to protect them from violations of human rights. Social work practitioners can take action towards economic rights by ensuring individuals have access to existing resources, conducting awareness-raising and consciousness-raising campaigns, lobbying against and resisting cuts in social assistance and social insurance programs, organizing communities for social justice, and promoting social entrepreneurship to promote self-sufficiency for those excluded from economic globalization (Staub-Bernasconi, 2007). Social workers can also promote rights-based approaches in their practice with low-income populations by developing a human rights culture in social work organizations, as well as other institutions such as schools, hospitals, and prisons. Social workers should also promote accountability through international human rights monitoring and reporting mechanisms. Practitioners can make use of international professional organizations such as the International Federation of Social Workers and International Association of Schools of Social Work Commissions on Human Rights. These international organizations consult with the UN and periodically issue statements and reports to UN agencies and human rights bodies. Legal advocacy is a powerful means of accountability; where enforced by law, rights-based claims can be made through public interest litigation (Midgley, 2007). Advocates have had success pursuing economic rights in South Africa where a community sued over water rights, in India where workers sued for employment rights and protections, and in Palestine where advocates are resisting Israeli settlements on the basis of the right to development (Midgley, 2007; Molyneux & Lazar, 2003; Moser & Norton, 2001).

Social workers can implement the right to development by advocating for policies and programs that address the rights of poor individuals, families, and communities. Social workers should examine development programs to ensure that none violate human rights in their pursuit of market-based economic growth. Policies designed for economic growth should be made sustainable, allowing for increased provision of resources for rights with improved structure of production and distribution. Social workers should work for rights-based reforms of national and international economic and development institutions.

For further reading on rights-based approaches to poverty

Centre for Development and Human Rights

An Indian research and advocacy organization founded by Arjun Sengupta, the first UN Special Rapporteur on Extreme Poverty, with resources for case studies. www.cdhr.org.in/

Special Rapporteur on Extreme Poverty and Human Rights

Annual reports, activities, policy statements, and more resources on poverty and human rights, including the 2013 report on the Participation of Persons Living in Poverty. www.ohchr.org/EN/Issues/Poverty/Pages/SRExtremePovertyIndex.aspx

UN practitioner's portal on human rights-based approaches to programming

Resources for budgeting, implementation, monitoring, and evaluation designed for practitioners to integrate rights-based approaches into a range of programs on women and children, development, disability, education, environment, health, emergencies, indigenous people, migrants and refugees, older adults, poverty, and more. http://hrbaportal.org/

UN Global Compact

A UN project partnering with private companies to bring human rights to global business. www.unglobalcompact.org/index.html

References

Abramovitz, M. (1988). *Regulating the lives of women: Social welfare policy from colonial times to the present.* Boston, MA: South End Press.

Androff, D. (2010a). Truth and reconciliation commissions (TRCs): An international human rights intervention and its connection to social work. *British Journal of Social Work, 40*(6), 1960–1977.

Androff, D. (2010b). 'To not hate': Reconciliation among victims of violence and participants of the Greensboro Truth and Reconciliation Commission. *Contemporary Justice Review, 13*(3), 269–285.

Androff, D. (2012a). Reconciliation in a community based restorative justice intervention: Victim assessments of the Greensboro Truth and Reconciliation Commission. *Journal of Sociology and Social Welfare, 39*(4), 73–96.

Androff, D. (2012b). Adaptations of truth and reconciliation commissions in the North American context: Local examples of a global restorative justice intervention. *Advances in Social Work: Special Issue on Global Problems and Local Solutions, 13*(2), 408–419.

Androff, D. (2012c). Narrative healing among victims of violence: The impact of the Greensboro Truth and Reconciliation Commission. *Families in Society, 93*(1), 10–16.

Androff, D. (in press). A case study of a grassroots truth and reconciliation commission from a community practice perspective. *Journal of Social Work.*

Annan, K. (2001). *3rd UN Conference on the Least Developed Countries, Brussels, Belgium, 14–20 May, 2001.* United Nations Office of the High Commissioner for Human Rights. Retrieved from: www.un.org/events/ldc3/conference/address/unhchr14_e.htm

Claude, R., & Weston, B. (Eds.). (2006). *Human rights in the world community: Issues and action* (3rd ed.). Philadelphia: University of Pennsylvania Press.

Despouy, L. (1996). *The realization of economic, social, and cultural rights: Final report on human rights and extreme poverty.* Special Rapporteur on Human Rights and Extreme Poverty. New York: United Nations.

Gatenio Gabel, S., & Kamerman, S. (2008). *Do conditional cash transfers work? The experience of the U.S. and developing countries.* Available at: www2.sofi.su.se/RC19/pdfpapers/Gatenio-Gabel_Kamerman_RC19_2008.pdf

Ife, J. (2012). *Human rights and social work: Towards rights-based practice* (3rd ed.). Cambridge: Cambridge University Press.

Jewell, J., Collins, K., Gargotto, L., & Dishon, A. (2009). Building the unsettling force: Social workers and the struggle for human rights. *Journal of Community Practice, 17*(3), 309–322.

Jones, A. (2005). The case of CARE International in Rwanda. In P. Gready & J. Ensor (Eds.), *Reinventing development: Translating rights-based approaches from theory into practice* (pp. 79–98). London: Zed Books.

Kindornay, S., Ron, J., & Carpenter, C. (2012). Rights-based approaches to development: Implications for NGOs. *Human Rights Quarterly, 34*(2), 472–506.

Lakoff, G. (2004). *Don't think of an elephant! Know your values and frame the debate.* White River Junction, VT: Chelsea Green.

Lindsey, D. (2003). *The welfare of children* (2nd ed.). Oxford: Oxford University Press.

Mapp, S. (2014). *Human rights and social justice in a global perspective* (2nd ed.). Oxford: Oxford University Press.

Marks, S. (2013). Poverty. In D. Moeckli, S. Shah, & S. Sivakumaran (Eds.), *International human rights law* (2nd ed., pp. 602–621). Oxford: Oxford University Press.

Midgley, J. (2007). Development, social development, and human rights. In E. Reichert (Ed.), *Challenges in human rights* (pp. 97–121). New York: Columbia University Press.

Midgley, J. (2010). Poverty, social assistance, and social investment. In J. Midgley & A. Conley (Eds.), *Social work and social development: Theories and skills for developmental social work*. Oxford: Oxford University Press.

Midgley, J. (2014). *Social development: Theory and practice.* Thousand Oaks, CA: Sage.

Midgley, J. & Conley, A. (Eds.). (2010). *Social work and social development: Theories and skills for developmental social work*. Oxford: Oxford University Press.

Molyneux, M., & Lazar, S. (2003). *Doing the rights thing: Rights-based development and Latin American NGOs*. London: ITDC.

Moser, C., & Norton, A. (2001). *To claim our rights: Livelihood, security, human rights, and sustainable development*. London: Overseas Development Institute.

Nickel, J. (2007). *Making sense of human rights*. Oxford: Wiley-Blackwell.

Nussbaum, M. (2011). *Creating capabilities: The human development approach*. Cambridge, MA: Belknap Press.

Offenheiser, R., & Holcombe, S. (2003). Challenges and opportunities in implementing a rights-based approach to development: An Oxfam-America perspective. *Nonprofit and Voluntary Quarterly, 32*(2), 268–301.

Pogge, T. (2011). Are we violating the rights of the world's poor? *Yale Human Rights & Development Law Journal, 14*(2), 1–33.

Reichert, E. (2011). *Social work and human rights: A foundation for policy* (2nd ed.). New York: Columbia University Press.

Sen, A. (1999). *Development as freedom*. New York: Alfred Knopf.

Sengupta, A. (2001). Right to development as a human right. *Economic and Political Weekly, 36*(27), 2527–2536.

Sengupta, A. (2006). The right to development. In R. Claude & B. Weston (Eds.), *Human rights in the world community: Issues and action* (3rd ed., pp. 249–258). Philadelphia: University of Pennsylvania Press.

Sengupta, A., Negi, A., & Basu, M. (Eds.). (2006). *Reflections on the right to development.* Thousand Oaks, CA: Sage.

Sherraden, M., & Stevens, J. (Eds.). (2010). *Lessons from SEED: A national demonstration of child development accounts*. St. Louis, MO: Center for Social Development, Washington University. Retrieved from: http://csd.wustl.edu/Publications/Documents/SEEDSynthesis_Final.pdf

Specht, H., & Courtney, M. (1994). *Unfaithful angles: How social work has abandoned its mission*. New York: Free Press.

Ssewamala, F., Sperber, E., Zimmerman, J., & Karimli, L. (2010). The potential of asset-based development strategies for poverty alleviation in Sub-Saharan Africa. *International Journal of Social Welfare, 19*(4), 433–443.

Staub-Bernasconi, S. (2007). Economic and social rights: The neglected human rights. In E. Reichert (Ed.), *Challenges in human rights: A social work perspective*. New York: Columbia University Press.

United Nations (UN). (1948, December 10). Universal Declaration of Human Rights. UN General Assembly. Retrieved from: www.un.org/Overview/rights.html

United Nations (UN). (1966). *International Covenant on Economic, Social, and Cultural Rights*. New York: Author. Retrieved from: www.ohchr.org/EN/ProfessionalInterest/Pages/CESCR.aspx

United Nations (UN). (1986). *Declaration on the Right to Development*. New York: Author. Retrieved from: www.un.org/documents/ga/res/41/a41r128.htm

United Nations (UN). (1993). *Vienna Declaration and Programme of Action.* World Conference on Human Rights. Retrieved from: www.ohchr.org/EN/ProfessionalInterest/Pages/Vienna.aspx

United Nations (UN). (2004). *Human rights and poverty reduction: A conceptual framework*. New York: United Nations Office of the High Commissioner for Human Rights. Retrieved from: www.ohchr.org/Documents/Publications/PovertyReductionen.pdf

United Nations (UN). (2008). *Claiming the MDGs: A human rights approach*. New York: UN High Commissioner for Human Rights. Retrieved from: www.ohchr.org/Documents/Publications/Claiming_MDGs_en.pdf

United Nations (UN). (2013). *The Millennium Development Goals Report 2013*. New York: Author. Retrieved from: www.un.org/millenniumgoals/pdf/report-2013/mdg-report-2013-english.pdf

United Nations Development Program (UNDP). (2003). *Poverty reduction and human rights: A practice note*. New York: Author. Retrieved from: www.undp.org/content/dam/aplaws/publication/en/publications/democratic-governance/dg-publications-for-website/poverty-reduction-and-human-rights-practice-note/HRPN_%28poverty%29En.pdf

United Nations Development Program (UNDP). (2007). *Human rights and the Millennium Development Goals: Making the link*. New York: Author. Retrieved from: www.undp.org/content/dam/aplaws/publication/en/publications/environment-energy/www-ee-library/water-governance/human-rights-and-the-millennium-development-goals-making-the-link/Primer-HR-MDGs.pdf

United Nations Development Program (UNDP). (2014). *Human Development Report 2014: Sustaining human progress: Reducing vulnerabilities and building resilience*. New York: Author. Retrieved from: http://hdr.undp.org/sites/default/files/hdr14-report-en-1.pdf

World Bank. (2013). *World Development Indicators 2013*. Washington, DC: Author. Retrieved from: http://databank.worldbank.org/data/download/WDI-2013-ebook.pdf

World Health Organization (WHO). (1995). *The World Health Report 1995: Bridging the gaps*. Geneva: Author.

Wronka, J. (2008). *Human rights and social justice: Social action and service for the helping and health professions*. Thousand Oaks, CA: Sage.

4

HUMAN RIGHTS-BASED APPROACHES TO CHILD WELFARE

Everyone begins life as a child; children have been called society's greatest resource for the future. The welfare of children is another area of central concern to the social work profession. This chapter identifies the implications of children's rights for social work practice with children. Social workers have been primarily concerned with child welfare, rather than children's rights. Despite this, a robust consensus on the human rights of children has emerged, and social workers should be aware of these developments.

Children's welfare, health, and survival is threatened worldwide. As small and dependent people, children often are among the most vulnerable and exploited groups (Mapp, 2014; UNDP, 2014). Over 6.6 million children die under the age of 5 each year, or 48 per 1,000 live births, mostly from preventable causes (Mapp, 2014; UNICEF, 2014). This is an estimated 18,000 child deaths every day. The global infant mortality rate is 35 per 1,000 live births. 15% of all newborns around the world suffer from low birth weight.

There are 150 million children who are orphans, over 17 million of whom are orphaned by AIDS (UNICEF, 2014). An estimated 15% of children globally suffer in child labor, about 215 million (Mapp, 2014). Eleven percent of female children are married by age 15; 34% by age 18. Only 65% of children under the age of 5 are registered. Twenty-one percent of women give birth before age 18.

More than one billion children suffer from lack of access to safe drinking water, adequate food, shelter, education, or health care (Mapp, 2014). One in seven children lives without any access to health services, or 270 million children. One in three children lives without adequate shelter, or 640 million children. One in five children lives without access to safe water, or 400 million children. About 1.4 million children die annually from a lack of access to safe drinking water and adequate sanitation.

Many, if not most, of these social indicators are linked to the prevalence of poverty among children. In the U.S., children are more likely to be poor than any other age group (Lindsey, 2003). Child poverty is a global problem, as are the associated violations of children's rights such as child labor, child sexual exploitation, and child soldiers (Mapp, 2014). The UN estimates that 121 million school-aged children, mostly girls, are not enrolled in school. Lack of access to education has been linked to child labor and poverty. School fees are prevalent across the Global South, and prevent many children from registering and attending school.

Children's rights, such as the right to education, are under attack in many places around the world. In 2014 the Nobel Peace Prize was awarded to children's rights activists Malala Yousafzai, a 17-year-old girl, and Kailash Satyarthi.

Traditional approaches to child welfare

Child welfare is unique as a field in which social work is more centrally involved than any other. This relates to the historical roots of the profession, as well as the degree of involvement; social work is more directly related to child welfare policy, administration and management, practice, and research than any other field of social work practice.

The profession of social work has been instrumental in several advancements in child welfare. In the 19th century, when most orphan children were placed in institutions, social workers pioneered reforms that led to the development of family care, resulting in the deinstitutionalization of dependent children (Sherraden et al., 2014). Early social work leadership in the prioritization of family care led to the expansion of foster care and kinship care models of child protection. Income support for needy families with dependent children was also influenced by social workers. In many countries, such as the U.S., social workers led the development of comprehensive child labor laws. Reductions in maternal and child mortality in the Global North, especially in the U.S. and Europe, were the result of social work interventions. Child abuse prevention and protection interventions were designed and led by social workers. Child protection systems vary globally; some states have robust systems of care while other states are still developing policies and systems to protect children.

However, many child welfare systems suffered from institutional racial and ethnic discrimination. Despite the best of intentions, social workers often implemented discriminatory state policy, reproducing patterns of oppression against poor and minority populations (Quadagno, 2004). The effects of such institutional racism can still be seen, for example, in the current racial disproportionalities of children in the child welfare and foster care systems, in which children of color are over-represented (Child Welfare Information Gateway, 2011).

In light of these accomplishments, and in spite of them, there remains a lot of room for improvement. Many child welfare systems are geared to focus upon child protection, not upon child well-being. Child investment strategies are increasingly important for social workers to incorporate into practice (Conley, 2010). Education also is a key area of social work involvement in child welfare. Finally, prevention is another growing area of social work practice with important benefits for children and families.

The human rights of children

All human rights apply to children, as they are human. Children's rights are contained in the core human rights documents, including the Universal Declaration of Human Rights, the International Convention on Civil and Political Rights, and the International Convention on Economic, Social and Cultural Rights. However, the human rights of children are most fully encapsulated in the 1989 Convention on the Rights of the Child (CRC) (UN, 1989).

Approaches to children's rights organize priorities in different ways. One common way, which applies to all populations, is the three Ps of protection, provision, and participation (Jones & Walker, 2011). Save the Children (2008) categorizes children's rights into four areas, the rights to survive, be safe, belong, and develop. UNICEF (2009) has developed the most well-known approach to children's rights, incorporating specific CRC articles into the categories of nondiscrimination, the best interest of the child, the rights to life, survival, and development, and finally respect for the views of the child.

Rights-based re-conceptualization of children

Human rights approaches re-conceptualize children from the perspective of the "whole child". In rights-based approaches, children are not seen as parental property, helpless objects of charity, adults-in-waiting, or passive dependents. A child is an individual and a member of a family and community with rights and responsibilities appropriate to their age and stage of development. Rights-based approaches to children, as exemplified by the Convention on the Rights of the Child, conceptualize and understand children as unique and deserving of special human rights consideration. In rights-based approaches, children are recognized as individuals who are among the most vulnerable, disempowered, and yet most important humans (UNICEF, 2014).

Children are among the most vulnerable humans. They start life completely dependent upon adults. Throughout much of their development, they remain dependent upon adults for their sustenance, protection, and guidance. Rights-based approaches recognize that members of children's primary family are ideal caregivers, i.e. parents, and further recognize that in the absence of family, society must fulfill this important function. Children are affected more deeply than any other social group by the actions or inactions of governments. Most public and social policies affect children – yet most policy fails to account for its impact upon children and thus can often have a negative impact upon children. Social changes, especially disruptive ones, bear a disproportionate impact on children. Many global trends, such as changing patterns of family structure, employment, migration, and reduced visions of state social welfare safety nets, have strong impacts on children. These are heightened in emergency cases of armed conflict or natural disasters.

Children are among the most disempowered humans. Children's experiences, perspectives, and viewpoints are rarely if ever heard in decision-making processes that affect them. Children are too young to vote or hold political office. Unless there are special efforts to include children's voices in local communities, schools, and homes, their perspective will be ignored on issues that affect them now or in the future.

Children are among the most important humans. The future success and welfare of any society is contingent upon the healthy development of children. Social conditions that limit child development hinder the economic development and social progress of any society. The consequences of failing to protect children's rights are significantly costly and overwhelmingly negative. Child development influences their subsequent life outcomes, and their contribution or cost to society.

The Convention on the Rights of the Child

In 1959 the UN signed the Declaration on the Rights of the Child, which was updated into the Convention on the Rights of the Child in 1989 (Mapp, 2014). This Convention has 140 signatories, 194 parties, and entered into force in 1990. The CRC contains provisions and principles from various legal systems and cultural traditions that represent universally agreed upon, non-negotiable standards and obligations for protecting children, meeting their basic needs, and maximizing their potential. The CRC recognizes that children aged 17 or under are especially vulnerable (Jones & Walker, 2011). It reinforces that children are entitled to the same human rights as all people, based on the principle of nondiscrimination, and adds additional protections for children. The CRC is comprehensive; it includes children's political, civil, economic, social, and cultural rights.

The guiding principle of the CRC is respect for "the best interests of the child", and is enshrined in Articles 3 and 18 which state that parents and other adults must always do what is best for children and young people (Jones & Walker, 2011). The CRC places responsibility for children's rights upon parents and states. Parents' paramount importance is affirmed in Article 5, which holds that parents have the best ability to promote children's rights consistent with their level of development. Article 4 speaks to the responsibility of governments to do everything they can to realize children's rights.

The CRC outlines a series of specific rights, including children's rights to an identity, participation, welfare, and protection from harm. The right to an identity is stated in Article 7, which specifies that all children have the right to birth registration and to a nationality (Tang & Lee, 2006). This right ensures that children have the documentation often necessary to access other rights such as education, employment, and voting. Identity documents also help to protect children against trafficking, conscription, and labor. This right requires a national policy and investment. UNICEF (2014) estimates that one third of global births, or 48 million children, go unregistered. This accounts for over half of all births in the Global South. Obstacles to birth registration include lack of national policies, documentation fees, lack of access to rural births, lack of birthright citizenship for children of immigrants (Malaysia and Thailand) and countries who do not register minority births (as is the case for Syrian Kurds, Baltic Russians, and Dominican Republican Haitians).

The CRC contains several articles that embody the human rights principle of participation. Participation is a fundamental human right for everyone, yet it is especially difficult to achieve children's participation given their dependent and developing status. Children's right to participation is qualified as "age-appropriate participation". Article 9 provides guidelines for custody courts to incorporate the voice of the child when determining where the child should live. Related to custody, children have the right to regular communication with both parents, provided this is in line with the best interest of the child. Article 12 says that children have the right to express themselves freely, and that their views must be given weight according to their age and maturity. Article 13 clarifies that children's right to freedom of expression includes the right to access to information and ideas. Article 14 confirms that children have the right to the freedom of religion, conscience, and of thought. Article 17 further states that although children have the right to information, they also have the right to be protected from harmful information.

The CRC also protects children's human right to survival and development. This includes their right to the best possible health and health care services (Article 24), the right to basic economic welfare, such as the rights to sufficient financial resources and an adequate standard of living in order for children to develop (Articles 26 and 27), and the right to free primary education, access to appropriate secondary education, and access to higher education (Article 28). Article 31 states that children have the right to rest, play, and to leisure, as part of their natural child and adolescent development. This right is critical to children's healthy development; children learn about the world and how to express themselves through play.

The CRC seeks to prevent harm to children. Child abuse and maltreatment is defined as harm that is proscribed, proximate, and preventable. The CRC prohibits societal abuse (child labor, child marriage, and child prostitution), physical maltreatment (abuse and neglect), sexual abuse (sexual contact and exposure to sexual stimuli), as well as nonphysical maltreatment (emotional mistreatment, parental substance abuse, fostering delinquency). Children's right to be free from abuse and exploitation is covered by several articles of the CRC, including Article 19, which states that children have the right to be protected from all forms of violence, abuse, neglect, and mistreatment; Article 20, stating that children have the right to special protections when they are separated from their parents; Article 32, which protects children from abuse, neglect, and economic and sexual exploitation; Article 34, which includes the right to protection from sexual exploitation, prostitution, and sexual abuse; Article 35, which states that children have the right to be protected from being removed from their family, sold, and trafficked; and Article 39, which states that governments have the responsibility to support and help children that have been hurt, abused, or exploited.

Child labor is given special attention in the CRC. It is prohibited under Article 32, which states that children have the right to be protected from economic exploitation, defined as work that is hazardous or interferes with the child's health and development, including physical, mental, spiritual, moral, or social development. An exception is made for "acceptable work" that assists in the development of a child, such as after school jobs and apprenticeships. Hazardous child labor is defined as street-work, agriculture work, domestic work, prostitution, and soldiering. Street-related forms of child labor are among the most visible, and include peddling and begging. The visibility of street children adds vulnerability through exposure to crime, rape, or police harassment. The majority of child labor is agricultural in nature, occurring on farms and in factories where children are exposed to dangerous machinery and harmful chemicals. Child domestic labor often occurs under hazardous and exploitative conditions and is accompanied by physical and sexual abuse. Prostitution includes the sale of children, child prostitution, and child pornography, and is further covered in the CRC's second optional protocol (UNICEF, 2009).

The CRC also protects the rights of children with special vulnerabilities (Jones & Walker, 2011). For example Article 22 guarantees refugee children the right to protection and humanitarian aid, and Article 23 guarantees disabled children the right to a full life and active participation in the community.

U.S. resistance to the CRC

The Convention on the Rights of the Child is among the world's most popular international human rights treaties. All but two of nation states in the world have signed it. These outliers are Somalia, which has lacked a functioning government for most of the time since the CRC's inception, and the U.S. The U.S. signed the CRC in 1995, under the Clinton administration, but has not submitted it to Congress for ratification (Mapp, 2014). Despite the near universal ratification of the CRC globally, the U.S. is unlikely to ratify the CRC due to cultural opposition, conflicts with existing law, and American federalism and exceptionalism (Whitaker, 2014).

American opponents to the CRC claim that the CRC threatens to undermine parental rights, if children's human rights are codified in law. Critics of the CRC aim to preserve parental authority over their children in the law, and are suspicious of measures to increase children's autonomy, particularly the CRC's implications for homeschooling, sex education, and even gun rights. Opponents also complain that the CRC contradicts current U.S. law; the CRC prohibits capital punishment for juveniles, which was legal in the U.S. before being deemed unconstitutional in 2005. The American government's system of federalism puts most policy pertaining to the human rights and welfare of children at the state level; the federal government is unlikely to impose CRC provisions upon individual states that bear the responsibility for protecting children's rights.

These are among the reasons that the U.S. lags behind in the ratification of many human rights agreements. The U.S.'s reluctance to ratify the CRC is also illustrative of the tension in balancing cultural norms and individual rights and relates to the larger debate between cultural relativism and universality. For example, whereas it is commonplace for American parents to sleep in separate rooms from their infants, this practice is regarded as neglectful and detrimental to child attachment and development in many cultures in the Global South. This divergence of what is considered appropriate parenting for healthy child development is why critics argue that the CRC's universal standards of children's human rights are inappropriate for the U.S.

Optional protocols to the Convention on the Rights of the Child

The CRC has three optional protocols. These include the Optional Protocol on the Rights of the Child on the Involvement of Children in Armed Conflict, the Optional Protocol on the Rights of the Child on the Sale of Children, Child Prostitution, and Child Pornography, and the Optional Protocol to the Convention on the Rights of the Child on a Communications Procedure.

The Optional Protocol on the Rights of the Child on the Involvement of Children in Armed Conflict was adopted in 2000 and entered into force in 2002 (UNICEF & Coalition to Stop the Use of Child Soldiers, 2003). It currently has 129 signatories and 155 state parties, including the U.S. This first Optional Protocol's purpose is to prevent anyone under the age of 18 from being recruited into the military or from serving in the armed forces with direct involvement in armed conflict and hostilities.

The Optional Protocol on the Rights of the Child on the Sale of Children, Child Prostitution, and Child Pornography was also adopted in 2000 and entered into force 2002 (UNICEF, 2009). It has 120 signatories and 167 parties, including the U.S. This second Optional Protocol focuses on the prohibition of the sale and trafficking of children, and child prostitution and pornography. UNICEF has publicized recommendations for rights-based implementation of the Optional Protocol and the development of child protection systems.

The Optional Protocol to the Convention on the Rights of the Child on a Communications Procedure was adopted in 2011 and entered into force in 2014. It currently has 45 signatories and 10 parties; the U.S. has not signed it. This third Optional Protocol enables children, groups of children, or their representatives to submit complaints about human rights violations and seek justice through the UN (NGO Group for the CRC, 2012). This Optional Protocol represents a major advancement of the principle of participation for children's rights; however, children can only access this complainant mechanism after all domestic legal remedies have been exhausted.

Committee on the Rights of the Child

Article 43 of the CRC created a Committee of the Rights of the Child, under the UN Office of the High Commissioner for Human Rights. The Committee is comprised of 18 experts to monitor the status of children's rights and implementation of the CRC and Optional Protocols among state parties (Tang & Lee, 2006). The Committee first met in 1991 (Claude, 2006). Article 45 of the CRC mandates UNICEF with a technical assistance role to provide consultation to the Committee and member states' reporting. The Committee periodically issues General Comments on the CRC which address special topics pertinent to children's rights and provide interpretation of various CRC provisions. The Committee has issued 14 such General Comments on topics ranging from education, migrating children, juvenile justice, children with disabilities, the impact of business, the right to play, and on the best interests of the child.

The Committee holds a biannual General Discussion Day on special topics to children's rights. Past discussion day topics include migration, incarcerated parents, the right to be heard, children without parental care, responsibilities of the state, indigenous children, private sector service providers, and violence against children. Discussion days solicit submissions from NGOs and working groups, and fact sheets and recommendations are prepared. Upcoming discussion day topics will include social media and access to justice and effective remedies.

The Committee also involves children in its work, honoring the principle of participation in a Child Participation Committee. The past chair, Millicent Atieno Orondo, was a 15-year-old girl from Kenya who addressed the UN General Assembly in 2007.

General Comment No. 5 of the Committee on the Rights of the Child

In 2003 the Committee on the Rights of the Child released General Comment No. 5, titled General Measures of Implementation of the Convention (UN, 2003). This general comment sought to expand upon Article 4 of the Convention on the Rights of the Child, which holds that states shall implement children's rights through legislative and administrative measures. This general comment has some practical implications for rights-based approaches, and builds upon the 2002 General Comment No. 2, on the role of Independent National Human Rights Institutions in the Protection and Promotion of the Rights of the Child. General Comment No. 5 affirms the CRC's priority of ensuring and maintaining child protection and care for children's well-being, relative to the rights and duties of parents. It also declares the indivisibility of children's civil and political rights with social, economic, and cultural rights as "inextricably intertwined" (UN, 2003, p. 3).

Right to education

The right to education is a vital component of children's rights. Education, from a rights-based perspective, has been named as essential for human dignity and the most valuable tool for personal empowerment (Claude, 2006; 2011). Education is a multi-faceted right linked to a variety of economic, political, and social rights – such as the right to full human development, economic employment, and self-sufficiency, and has been identified as a prerequisite for participation in modern life.

Education has been highlighted for its importance in realizing all other human rights (Claude, 2006). Human rights advocates emphasize human rights education as education towards a human rights culture. The right to education is contained in Article 26 of the Universal Declaration with three goals, the full development of the human personality, the promotion of tolerance, and the maintenance of peace. The rationale for including a right to education in the UDHR was the prevention of future war, conflict, and violence through the promotion of a culture of respect for human rights. Education is not considered to be value-neutral, but a means to promote a holistic view of human nature as free, social, and entitled to participate in decision-making processes. A core assumption of the UDHR is that states who respect human rights will be less likely to go to war against each other, resulting in a more peaceful and stable world.

Right to a family

Another important right to note is children's right to their own family. The forced removal and transfer of children from their families and communities is considered to be a category of genocide. The fifth category under the Convention on the Prevention and Punishment of the Crime of Genocide states that the removal of children and transfer to another group constitutes genocide, commonly referred to as cultural genocide. This was the case of forced schooling of indigenous children in North America and Australia.

Article 9 of the CRC contains the rights of children to parental care, Articles 20 and 21 protect the rights of children without parental care, and Articles 10 and 12 specify the rights of children to family reunification. This is particularly salient for migrant and refugee children separated from their families. The Committee on the Rights of the Child's General Discussion Day of 2012 addressed separation of children and parents through immigration enforcement policies of detention and deportation. The Committee issued a report detailing migrant children's rights to a family life, specifically for detention and deportation.

Case study of a rights-based approach to child welfare

Many NGOs promoting international child welfare across the Global South have adopted rights-based approaches. Some of these include UNICEF, Children's Rights Information Network, Childwatch International Research Network, PLAN International, Street Kids International, Coalition to Stop the Use of Child Soldiers, CARE International and Save the Children (Lansdown, 2005; Save the Children, 2008). This section draws a case study of rights-based approaches to child welfare from one of these. This chapter's case study comes from an international NGO's program in one African country that is attempting a transformation from a humanitarian aid to a human rights-based organization.

CARE International – Rwanda

CARE International (CARE) originated in the U.S. after World War II to deliver humanitarian aid to Europe (Jones, 2005). Now CARE conducts a range of anti-poverty initiatives in 87 countries through more than 900 projects (www.care.org). In the late 1990s, CARE began a process of reflection and dialogue at its highest levels on how to integrate human rights into all its work. This led to a period of experimentation with rights-based approaches in the field.

Rwanda is a small country in the Great Lakes region of Africa. This former European colony has suffered from an infamous genocide and ongoing violence and destabilization throughout the region, including the neighboring Congo. Despite significant progress since the genocide, many challenges remain for rights in Rwanda, including a limited civil society and lack of public participation, which can result in a tendency toward acquiescence to authority.

CARE began working in Rwanda in 1984. Its office is staffed mostly by Rwandans. It has been deeply involved in the post-genocide reconstruction, and worked extensively with orphans of violence and HIV/AIDS and other vulnerable children. Its main emphasis is upon poverty alleviation, and it has attempted to incorporate a rights-based approach to its programming to realize the rights of Rwanda's poor and vulnerable. Its services include psychosocial support to orphans and vulnerable children, while working on a larger agenda of promoting good governance and civil society. Since the genocide, CARE in Rwanda has been working to mainstream a human rights perspective in order to maximize its impact and achieve social transformation to prevent a return to violence. A major focus of CARE Rwanda's program is to provide psychosocial support to orphans and vulnerable children (CARE, 2011).

CARE views human rights as holistic entitlements that enable people to live to their full potential with dignity (Jones, 2005). In their transition from a service-oriented organization towards a rights-based approach, the provision of services and aid shifted from being their program's end to instead a means to an end; delivering aid is a way to realize human rights. CARE Rwanda incorporated a human rights perspective into every element of their program design, practice, and evaluation. CARE Rwanda fostered staff investment in rights-based approaches through human rights education, linking human rights to traditional Rwanda cultural values, and encouraging discussion. CARE Rwanda's rights-based approach included community mapping, participatory action planning, social theater and radio, awareness raising and community education, dialogue on social conditions, and legal services.

Nkundabana Initiative for Psychosocial Support (NIPS)

An estimated 48% of the Rwandan population is illiterate, a violation of their right to education. CARE Rwanda uses a community-based program led by community members to teach literacy, life skills, and vocational training to poor children, especially girls. This is similar to a promotora approach, but in Rwanda it is called Nkundabana. The program has increased school attendance among vulnerable youth, and resulted in positive child protection outcomes (CARE, 2011). The project has been expanded to include the development of parent-teacher associations, early child development, and child health measures against pneumonia, malaria, and diarrhea.

CARE Rwanda serves about 2,250 child-headed households across the country (Jones, 2005). These children identify to CARE the children-headed households, where the oldest sibling or child in the home is less than 21 years old. Nkudabana, or indigenous peer leaders, are nominated by children, who as volunteers make home visits and give psychosocial support to children without adult support (Pells, 2010). The children receive extensive education on HIV/AIDS and other health topics, human rights and empowerment, and social and peer support organizations. The children and Nkundabana present their perspective at regular meetings with authorities.

The NIPS program yielded a positive shift in the community perception of children, particularly orphaned children and their rights, which relates to the principle of dignity (Pells, 2010). NIPS led to positive outcomes such as reduced resentment, increased local ownership, and sustainability. The NIPS program is an example of the rights-based principle of participation (Pells, 2010). Facilitating the participation of the Nkundabana required investment of CARE Rwanda resources into youth participants, as well as giving programmatic control and leadership to participants. Such programs need community education to build support and acceptance; many parents were jealous of NIPS without realizing the program was specifically designed to target orphans (Pells, 2010). This relates to the need for transparency; children and community members need to have clear understanding of the selection criteria and of the program expectations. There was some confusion among child participants that they would receive houses, when that was never a key aspect of the program. Incorporating child feedback is also important; participants suggested reforming eligibility to include children with parents who might be just as vulnerable if not more due to poverty or substance abuse.

Rights-based practice principles

CARE Rwanda implemented the rights-based principles for practice. Human rights were seen as the way to enable people to live with dignity, promote self-determination, and to support poor people's control over their own lives. CARE adjusted its traditional view of people as clients and beneficiaries to seeing the people they serve as rights-holders. CARE Rwanda affirmed nondiscrimination by focusing on vulnerable Rwandans whose rights had been systematically violated. The principle of participation was enacted when they incorporated the involvement of children in the design and delivery of NIPS and using local youth to be ambassadors and initiate community change.

CARE Rwanda implemented transparency in its analysis of the root causes of poverty as a violation of human rights. They adapted a tool from UNICEF to create a new assessment mechanism (Jones, 2005). The Causal-Responsibility Analysis (CRA) begins with identifying a specific right that is being violated, then analyzes the causal factors of the violation, and assesses the party who is responsible for maintaining the right. This links human rights violations to their underlying cause and the responsibility and capabilities of duty-bearers. Its analysis goes beyond quantitative or qualitative measures that describe a snapshot, overview, or individual experience of a problem to an analysis of the rights deprivation (Jones, 2005). The causal-responsibility analysis is a concrete method to work towards the principle of transparency in practice and push programs beyond provision of social services to socio-political action through rights-based analysis and design. The results lead to positive actions that can be implemented by program staff, participants, and duty-bears in order to realize the violated right. The CARE Rwanda program used the CRA tool to move beyond its traditional service provision, characterized by short-term emergency responsive measures, to longer term social and political action addressing the factors that created the need for services. This contributed to not only meeting the immediate need of children orphaned by HIV/AIDS, but also addressed their dignity and self-worth. Instead of stopping once the immediate suffering of the orphans was ameliorated, CARE Rwanda continued to work on the deeper issues of discrimination, ignorance, exploitation, and exclusion that impact the orphans' long-term well-being. For example, using a rights-based assessment CARE Rwanda identified obstacles preventing children from accessing their right to education, and developed a strategy to raise awareness of the government's universal primary education policy, prevent child labor, and promote family planning and access to reproductive health services. Another analysis identified factors relating to discrimination and social exclusion of certain groups of children, and resulted in action steps to promote tolerance among the population, address the stereotyping and discriminatory beliefs, and create access to local public officials and resources.

CARE Rwanda also developed a participatory program evaluation tool to conduct rights-based monitoring for bottom-up accountability. This consisted of regular forums for CARE program participants, the children from child-headed households, to give feedback and criticism of the program. Each session was conducted in safe settings and began with a staff update about how the last round of feedback was incorporated. Then a limited set of questions was used to gather additional feedback and critique. These questions complement data collection measures of child well-being and focus on rights-based issues of discrimination, protection, and participation. Finally, space is made for children to raise their own, self-identified, issues on their own terms. The children's input was seen as an essential piece of monitoring and is incorporated into ongoing program design and overall project direction. This mechanism emphasizes accountability, and CARE committed itself to responding to all feedback. By making the organization accountable to the voice of children, CARE effectively began to share power and give a measure of control to the child participants.

Rights-based approach to social work practice with children

Social work practice can incorporate the rights-based practice principles of dignity, non-discrimination, participation, transparency, and accountability. Rights-based approaches affirm the inherent human dignity of children by recognizing them as rights-holders, not as objects of charity. The human dignity of children relates to their best interest. The Convention on the Rights of the Child and child welfare practitioners are guided by the principle of the best interests of the child. This requires that practitioners systematically consider the impact of their actions, decisions, and programs upon children, both directly and indirectly. Dignity and the best interest of the child mean protecting children's right to life, survival, and development. A rights-based understanding of child development encompasses physical, mental, spiritual, moral, psychological, and social development.

In order to fully implement nondiscrimination, practitioners should work for legislative, administrative, budgetary, and educational reforms. Non-discrimination does not necessarily mean identical treatment for all children. Social work practice should balance realizing the rights of all children with also attending to special needs of disadvantaged populations of children. Nondiscrimination in child welfare requires social workers to ascertain which individual and groups of children are vulnerable to discrimination, and identify when discrimination is occurring and against whom. Social workers must also take action to combat the underlying causes of discrimination.

The principle of children's participation means that social workers should support children's right to express their views freely in all matters affecting them. Social workers should actively include children in the promotion, protection, and monitoring of children's rights. Although active participation in voting is limited to people who are 18 years old, children should be encouraged to participate in political forums. Securing children's participation may involve consultations with children. Consultations should be consistent and ongoing, as opposed to singular one-time affairs. Children's participation in social work practice can be met through regular direct contact between children and child welfare practitioners. Social workers must ensure that consultations go beyond tokenistic listening towards the realization of children's rights. Specific populations of children may need to be consulted at different times, for example children in foster care should be consulted when considering reforms to adoption and foster care policies and programs.

Transparency in rights-based approaches to child welfare includes research, training, and education with accurate knowledge to inform social work practice. Rights-based child welfare indicators are necessary for identifying discrimination, evaluating programs, assessing progress of implementation, and for reporting requirements under the CRC. Social workers should develop social indicators related to children's rights contained in the CRC (McNamara, 2013). Social workers should apply research methods that incorporate children's views and input as they are in the best position to indicate if their rights are being realized and if their voices are being heard in their families, schools, and communities. Evaluation efforts should emphasize interviews with children, participatory research methods with children, and using children as researchers. Paramount in child-related research is their protection from exploitation through research processes and through the dissemination of information. Further research should evaluate respectful approaches for practitioners to conduct child and adolescent research, based on children's right to express opinions on matters affecting them and express their views in the way they wish. Social workers should strive to make research accessible to children, fulfilling their right to information.

Rights-based social work practice with children requires extensive training and capacity building for social workers. Social workers, in turn, should work to train government officials, the judiciary, teachers, community leaders, police and juvenile detention staff, and parents on children's rights. Trainings should cover children's rights, attitudes and practices of child welfare, cultural context of children's rights, and emphasizing children as rights-holders. Trainings should also be incorporated into school curricula at all levels so that capacity building can occur with children themselves, keeping with the principle of participation, and tied to larger efforts at human rights education. Learning about human rights should be a lifelong process, grounded in everyday life experiences, especially for children. Children should learn about human rights from examples of how they are implemented in families, in schools, and in communities. Social workers should link awareness-raising about children's rights to processes of social change and transformation via interactive, dialogic, and participatory formats. Social workers should disseminate information on children's rights widely and in child-accessible formats, to inform policymaking and generate public engagement. Human rights monitoring reports and documents on children's rights, prepared by states and NGOs, should be disseminated and discussed in order to maximize their impact on facilitating an atmosphere supportive of children's rights and to positively impact children's lives.

Accountability for children's rights should result a shift in perception of children's social status, and prioritizing children's rights politically with sensitivity to the impact of policies on children (Wronka, 2008). Social workers should advocate and engage in policy practice to promote policies that uphold the rights of children, including child care, maternity leave, and family policies that promote work and prevent poverty. Social workers should advocate for children to have universal access to high quality, evidence-based social services on a sustainable basis. This requires social workers to aim to mainstream children's rights into economic and development policies and programs.

Social workers should advocate for legislation that is consistent with the CRC. Social workers should develop and deliver policies, services, and programs to implement children's rights. Social workers should work to create and support child-centered organizations, structures, and activities, such as children's rights units in government, administrative, and legislative committees on children, child impact analyses, children's budgets, "state of the children's rights" reports, and coalitions on children's rights. Social workers should hold accountable not just public but also private child care and child welfare actors through regulation and monitoring.

Social workers can conduct child impact assessments and evaluations for ongoing monitoring, in collaboration with NGOs, state parties, academic institutions, professional organizations, youth groups, media organizations, and independent human rights institutions.

Social workers can promote state accountability for children's rights through budgetary analysis of investments in children's rights, raising publicity about the state's responsibility to fulfilling rights to the maximum extent of available resources. Social workers can publish children's budgets that highlight and detail both direct and indirect spending on children. Making children visible in budgets is the essence of administrative planning for children's economic, social, and cultural rights, and indicates state priorities of children's rights. Incorporating children's rights into budgets can ensure that children, as the most vulnerable members of society, are protected from the negative aspects of economic cycles and policies including recessions as well as the austerity programs designed in their wake. This is also relevant to structural adjustment programs and states transitioning to market economies, who may be experiencing distorted development in the midst of overall economic progress. Social development policies are instrumental in ensuring investments in children's rights.

Legal protections are especially necessary for children's rights, given children's dependency. Social workers should facilitate child-friendly mechanisms for access to legal information, advice, advocacy services, and tools for their self-advocacy. This must include access to independent complaint mechanisms. Upon determination of the violation of children's rights, children should be provided redress such as compensation, physical and psychological recovery, rehabilitation, and reintegration.

For further reading on rights-based approaches to child welfare

Child Soldiers International

Formerly Coalition to Stop the Use of Child Soldiers, this NGO was established by leading human rights and humanitarian organizations to develop the Optional Protocol to the Convention on the Rights of the Child on the Involvement of Children in Armed Conflict, now focused on its implementation.
www.child-soldiers.org/

Children of the Forest

An NGO working with stateless children on the Thai border.
http://childrenoftheforest.org/

Childwatch International Research Network

A global network of institutions conducting child research promoting child rights and monitoring the Convention on the Rights of the Child.
www.childwatch.uio.no/

Plan International

International NGO promoting the rights of children in poverty.
https://plan-international.org/

REPLACE Campaign

An NGO raising awareness about children's rights and the risks of institutionalization, focused on moving children from orphanages into families.
www.replace-campaign.org/

Save the Children

An international NGO promoting child rights.
www.savethechildren.net/

UNICEF

The UN Children's Fund, international child-rights organization.
www.unicef.org/

References

CARE International. (2011). *Rwanda fact sheet*. Retrieved from: www.care.org/sites/default/files/documents/rwanda-fact-sheet-2011.pdf

Child Welfare Information Gateway. (2011). *Addressing racial disproportionality in child welfare*. Washington, DC: U.S. Department of Health and Human Services, Children's Bureau. Retrieved from: www.childwelfare.gov/pubPDFs/racial_disproportionality.pdf

Claude, R. (2006). The right to education and human rights education. In R. Claude & B. Weston (Eds.), *Human rights in the world community: Issues and action* (3rd ed., pp. 211–223). Philadelphia: University of Pennsylvania Press.

Claude, R. (2011). A letter to my colleagues, students, and readers of *Human Rights Quarterly*. *Human Rights Quarterly, 33*(2), 578–585.

Conley, A. (2010). Childcare: Welfare or investment? *International Journal of Social Welfare, 19*(2), 173–181.

Jones, A. (2005). The case of CARE International in Rwanda. In P. Gready & J. Ensor (Eds.), *Reinventing development?: Translating rights-based approaches from theory into practice* (pp. 79–98). London: Zed Books.

Jones, P., & Walker, G. (Eds.). (2011). *Children's rights in practice*. Los Angeles: Sage.

Lansdown, G. (2005). *Benchmarking progress in adopting and implementing child rights programming*. London: Save the Children. Retrieved from: www.crin.org/docs/resources/publications/hrbap/CRP_benchmark_study.pdf

Lindsey, D. (2003). *The welfare of children* (2nd ed.). Oxford: Oxford University Press.

Mapp, S. (2014). *Human rights and social justice in a global perspective: An introduction to international social work* (2nd ed.). New York: Oxford University Press.

McNamara, P. (2013). Rights-based narrative research with children and young people conducted over time. *International Social Work, 12*(2), 135–152.

NGO Group for the CRC. (2012). *Advocacy toolkit: Campaign for the ratification of the third Optional Protocol to the CRC on a communications procedure*. Retrieved from: http://ratifyop3crc.org/wp-content/uploads/2014/03/Advocacy_toolkit_May-2012-short-version-EN.pdf

Pells, K. (2010). 'No one ever listens to us': Challenging obstacles to the participation of children and young people in Rwanda. In B. Percy-Smith & N. Thomas (Eds.), *A handbook of children and young people's participation: Perspectives from theory and practice* (pp. 196–203). London: Routledge.

Quadagno, J. (2004). *The color of welfare.* New York: Oxford University Press.

Save the Children. (2008). Toolkit: Child rights situation analysis. Stockholm: Save the Children Sweden. Retrieved from: www.crin.org/docs/Child_Rights_Situation_Analysis_Final%5B1%5D.pdf

Sherraden, M., Stuart, P., Barth, R., Kemp, S., Lubben, J., Hawkins, J., . . . Catalano, R. (2014). *Grand accomplishments in social work.* Grand Challenges for Social Work Initiative, Working Paper No. 2. Baltimore, MD: American Academy of Social Work and Social Welfare. Retrieved from: http://aaswsw.org/wp-content/uploads/2013/12/FINAL-Grand-Accomplishments-sb-12-9-13-Final.pdf

Tang, K., & Lee, J. (2006). Global social justice for older people: The case for an international convention on the rights of older people. *British Journal of Social Work, 36*(7), 1135–1150.

UNICEF & Coalition to Stop the Use of Child Soldiers. (2003). *Guide to the Optional Protocol on the Involvement of Children in Armed Conflict.* New York: Author. Retrieved from: www.unicef.org/sowc06/pdfs/option_protocol_conflict.pdf

United Nations (UN). (1989). *Convention on the Rights of the Child.* New York: Author. Retrieved from: www.ohchr.org/en/professionalinterest/pages/crc.aspx

United Nations (UN). (2003). *General Comment No. 5. General Measures on Implementation of the Convention on the Rights of the Child.* New York: UN Committee on the Rights of the Child. Retrieved from: http://daccess-dds-ny.un.org/doc/UNDOC/GEN/G03/455/14/PDF/G0345514.pdf?OpenElement

United Nations Children's Fund (UNICEF). (2009). *Handbook on the Optional Protocol on the Sale of Children, Child Prostitution, and Child Pornography.* Florence, Italy: UNICEF Innocenti Research Centre. Retrieved from: www.unicef-irc.org/publications/pdf/optional_protocol_eng.pdf

United Nations Children's Fund (UNICEF). (2014). *The State of the World's Children 2014 in Numbers: Every child counts – Revealing disparities, advancing children's rights.* New York: Author. Retrieved from: www.unicef.org/sowc2014/numbers/documents/english/SOWC2014_In Numbers_28 Jan.pdf

United Nations Development Program (UNDP). (2014). *Human Development Report 2014: Sustaining human progress: Reducing vulnerabilities and building resilience.* New York: Author. Retrieved from: http://hdr.undp.org/sites/default/files/hdr14-report-en-1.pdf

Whitaker, K. (2014). Social justice and the politics of children's rights. In M. Austin (Ed.), *Social justice and social work* (pp. 139–148). Thousand Oaks, CA: Sage.

Wronka, J. (2008). *Human rights and social justice: Social action and service for the helping and health professions.* Thousand Oaks, CA: Sage.

5

HUMAN RIGHTS-BASED APPROACHES WITH OLDER ADULTS

Human aging represents a triumph of humanity and the overcoming of myriad afflictions that have caused mortality for millennia. Advances in health, preventative medicine, family planning, and sanitation have driven increases in human life expectancy resulting in a massive global demographic transformation (Hokenstad & Roberts, 2012). Human aging presents new challenges as well as opportunities.

The demographic tsunami of global aging

In 1950 it is estimated that there were only 200 million people over 60 years old. In 2000, 10% of the world's population was over 60 (Mukherjee, 2009). By 2006 this increased to 700 million, with 64% in the Global South (Huenchuan & Rodriguez-Pinero, 2011). This was an increase of over 50% from 2000. Demographic estimates project even more dramatic transformations; by 2050, 2 billion people, over 20% of the world's population will be age 60 or older, with an estimated 80% in the Global South (Hokenstad & Roberts, 2012). The ratio of older adults to the rest of the population in the Global South was 1 in 12 in 2005, and is expected to increase to 1 in 5 by 2050. The worldwide average life expectancy is estimated to add 11 years by 2050, and the population of older adults over 80 is expected to grow the most.

The increase in older adults is linked to dramatic population growth rates. Overall, the population growth rate is 1.1%, but for older adults it is 2.6%, and in the Global South it is 3.3%. The population growth rate of adults over 80 worldwide is 3.9%, while in the Global South it is 5%. Regional impacts will be significant. Among adults over 60 in Africa, the growth rate is a stunning 310%. Older adults in Latin America and the Caribbean have a population growth rate three to five times greater than the total (Huenchuan & Rodriguez-Pinero, 2011). Over half of the growth in older adults is expected to occur in Asia; China and India may have

600 million older adults in 2020 (Mukherjee, 2009). Countries such as Colombia and Malaysia may see their aging populations increase by 200%.

Conceptions of aging

Aging brings both fullness and loss, varying by culture, generation, and historical moment. "Old" is thought to mean the loss of instrumental and functional capacity necessary for independence and self-determination (Huenchuan & Rodriguez-Pinero, 2011). Aging is a multifaceted process determined by social and cultural factors in addition to biological functions. Old age is a socially constructed identity, similar to childhood and adolescence (Fredvang & Biggs, 2012). A hundred years ago, in much of the world, 40 years was considered old. Today the chronological age used by the majority of nations is 60 for the purpose of legislation, yet it is growing ever more difficult to pinpoint an age at which one becomes "old".

Scholars have identified three lenses to view age: chronological, social, and physiological. Social policies tend to refer to people's chronological age in typically defining eligibility at 60 or 65 years of age. The decline of physical and functional capacity that occurs over time to the human body is understood as physiological aging. Social age refers to how a biologically based category of people are framed by subjective perceptions resulting in a combination of how old someone feels and how old others perceive them to be. Class, race and ethnicity, gender, and other social factors combine with genetics to constitute one's "social age". Social norms about aging revolve around older adults' health, capacity for work, need for social support, and conflict with younger generations.

Older adults are defined relative to social norms, which tend to be biased towards youth. Most institutions are oriented towards a normative standard of people of working age. Older adults, traditionally falling outside that category, face exclusion from these structures. Most interventions are designed from this perspective, and manage or maintain the social exclusion of older adults.

Consequences associated with aging

Although aging can bring many opportunities, it is often associated with problems of health, quality of life, elder abuse, discrimination, exclusion, and isolation. Health risks increase with age. Declining infectious and acute diseases and the concomitant declining birth and death rates have caused an increase in chronic degenerative and incapacitating disease among the aging of the population (Huenchuan & Rodriguez-Pinero, 2011). Older adults are also vulnerable to physical abuse, violence, and exploitation. Health concerns, including those of mental health, such as dementia, place older adults at risk for violations of self-determination, privacy, information, and mobility (Fredvang & Biggs, 2012). Health care for older adults raise questions of quality of life.

Age discrimination, the specific prejudice and stereotyping of persons based on their age, is one of the central problems faced by older adults as it can limit all their other human rights (Fredvang & Biggs, 2012; Huenchuan & Rodriguez-Pinero, 2011; Tang & Lee, 2006). Age discrimination entails the risk of loss of economic resources and poverty, invisibility and exclusion from political agendas, and power-lessness. Ageism can be both interpersonal and institutional. Most anti-ageism laws are limited to age discrimination in employment.

Older adults disproportionately suffer from poverty (ILO, 2014). Older adults' lack of a minimum standard of living results from widespread inadequate social protection and declining employment and productivity. This can be exacerbated by disability, mandatory retirement ages, gender restrictions on inheritance laws, and financial exploitation. Forty-eight percent of all older adults do not receive a pension; of those who do receive a pension, many are inadequate. The issue of older adults in poverty is exacerbated in the Global South where an estimated 36% of older adults do not receive a pension providing income security.

These factors often result in the social exclusion of older adults. Older adults often face community or social isolation; many lack access to food, water, and services. Traditional family support is declining in many countries (Kollapan, 2008). This has been attributed to the impact of globalization, changing and rearranging cultural and social norms and practices (Mukherjee, 2009). These have diminished the status of older adults and furthered their social exclusion.

Conclusion

Global aging will be felt by both the Global North and the Global South, with significant impact upon social, economic, and political structures (Huenchuan & Rodriguez-Pinero, 2011). The number and proportion of adults aged 60 years and older will continue to grow. More of the adult population will be older adults; declining fertility rates increase the portion of older adults. Older adults are getting older; the fastest growing age group is adults 80 years and older. The aging of the population is gendered; most older adults are women. Of adults over 80 years old, women outnumber men by nearly 2 to 1. These changes will increase pressure upon public policy, social services, and social workers. In the Global North, the political impact of the demographic surge that followed World War II has already begun to strain the capacity of social service programs and professionals, resulting in recent debates surrounding entitlement reform, public spending, and privatization. However, the issues facing older adults, from poverty to discrimination, have not played a major part of domestic or international policy agendas (Tang & Lee, 2006).

Existing safety nets for older adults are virtually nonexistent or weak in many places across the Global South. The lack of social protection, shortage of savings due to low wages throughout many years of work, and increased health problems and disabilities limit their self-sufficiency. The gendered nature of aging, i.e. the predominance of older adults who are women, signifies even greater social exclusion based on sexism and gender-based discrimination (Tang & Lee, 2006; UN, 2010). The situation of older women is reinforced by their care-giving responsibilities, such as caring for grandchildren or sick and disabled relatives.

The responsibility of care giving falls primarily on women (Fredvang & Biggs, 2012). In Africa, the HIV/AIDS epidemic has both increased the care-giving responsibilities of older adults and weakened family cohesion that nurtures older adults (Kollapan, 2008). This tremendous demographic change is driving the need to examine and develop rights-based approaches for older adults.

Traditional approaches to older adults

Social and economic patterns since industrialization have connected social status to economic productivity and prioritized individualism over family and community needs (Giunta, 2010). Old age has become seen as a time of diminished economic productivity and diminished status. As older adults shift from productive economic actors to unproductive dependents, they experience a loss of social identity. Urbanization fragmens families and social networks; older adults become more socially isolated, their health and mental health worsens, and they are exposed to greater risk of abuse and exploitation.

Traditional policy and practice interventions for older adults have focused on the problems associated with old age such as reduced income, decreased autonomy, and the loss of social role and identity (Huenchuan & Rodriguez-Pinero, 2011). This is based on a Western conception of aging as a time of increased economic, physical, and social needs, and has shaped policy measures to focus on supplementing these areas, in contrast to empowering adults to attain the highest possible standard of living.

The limitation of these approaches is that they regard older adults as a problem to be solved, a burden upon their families, workers, future generations, and society at large (Tang & Lee, 2006). This is especially the case in the Global North where interventions are heavily influenced by the medical model which emphasizes diagnosis of illness, treatment of physical defect or harm, and overall a reductionist view towards human and social issues.

Many states expanded social welfare programs to older adults in the decades following World War II, strengthening intergenerational compacts through contributory schemes (Guseilo, Curl & Hokenstad, 2004). Recent retrenchments and attacks against traditional welfare program and statist approaches have jeopardized these gains. Neoliberal approaches to social welfare have curtailed policies and programs supporting older adults (Tang & Lee, 2006). In addition to threatening support for expanding programs that aid older adults (in favor of privatization) this dynamic has kept central an economic focus to the debate, neglecting social, health, and even rights-based approaches to older adults for a perspective that places "retirement" as the primary concern for older adults. This is despite the unparalleled success of programs such as social security in the U.S. lifting older adults from poverty; prior to social security, to become old was synonymous with becoming poor. Now older adults in the U.S. have the lowest incidence of poverty.

Global aging threatens to overwhelm current policies, practices, and programs (Hokenstad & Choi, 2012). Social workers are inadequately prepared, in both training and funding, to meet the challenges of global aging (Mukherjee, 2009). The demand for gerontological social workers will increase, and there will be further need to train professionals (Hokenstad & Roberts, 2012). In light of this, what strategies and practices should social workers adopt, promote, and implement to address global aging? Predominant discourse on responding to global aging centers mainly on the Global North; therefore it is necessary to discuss the Global South as well, since global aging will be more transformational to societies there (Mukherjee, 2009).

In the Global North, faced with declining family and community support, older adults exercised their political rights by forming advocacy organizations, such as AARP (formerly the American Association of Retired Persons), which has become the largest political lobby in the U.S. (Mukherjee, 2009). AARP and related organizations such as SeniorNet have effectively lobbied for the rights of older adults on policy issues such as mandatory retirements, age caps on drivers licenses, and affordable health care and prescription medications. In the Global South, traditional social structures supporting older adults, such as family and community care and co-residence, have meant less government intervention. Policies and programs for older adults in the Global South have remained underdeveloped. The lack of state resources and the pressures of overpopulation have caused them to rely upon existing social capital for support (Mukherjee, 2009). However, the acceleration of economic globalization increasingly disrupts traditional structures and diminishes social capital. For example as economic opportunity manifests in cities, urbanization increases and co-residence decreases. Older adults face declining social support, and simultaneously decreased economic opportunity as many new jobs brought by globalization are inaccessible to older adults (Mukherjee, 2009). Women, who provide most care for older adults, are benefiting from economic globalization through economic participation in the new labor markets yet are able to provide less care in family settings. China's 2013 law mandating that children visit their parents annually, resulting in at least one prosecution so far, is an example of the way that rapid economic growth can disrupt traditional family structures and how states may attempt to legislate the preservation of familial relations for older adults (Wong, 2013).

Contemporary approaches to older adults over-emphasize health and retirement rather than active participation and positive contribution. Taken together, neoliberal reductions in social welfare programs and promotion of free market approaches represent challenges to the welfare of older adults (Tang & Lee, 2006). In this context, rights-based approaches for older adults are very important to explore and to develop.

The human rights of older adults

Although all human rights are the right of older adults, there is no comprehensive international human rights agreement specifically addressing older adults (Rodriguez-Pinzon & Martin, 2003). Older adults remain a vulnerable population in lack of an international legal instrument to protect their rights. The human rights of children and older adults are similar in that they are only rights dependent upon the passage of time and a certain age. Children's rights, considered more developed as evidenced by the CRC, may yield insight into the process of articulating the rights of older adults.

Universal Declaration of Human Rights (UDHR)

The human rights of older adults stem, as do everyone's, from the 1948 UDHR (UN, 1948), and have been refined in the 1966 ICCPR and ICESCR. Article 2 of the UDHR prohibits discrimination and contains the principle of universality; all human rights apply to older adults because human rights are universal and apply to everyone. Non-discrimination is a fundamental component of rights-based approaches, and most international human rights documents prohibit discrimination against people on the basis of certain characteristics. In Article 2, the UDHR does not specify age in its prohibition of discrimination on the basis of "race, color, sex, language, religion, political or other opinion, national or social origin, property, birth or other status". Although age is not listed, there is consensus that these categories are not limiting, and that grounds for discrimination extends beyond this list (UN, 1989). Therefore the principle of non-discrimination is a broad and universal principle extending beyond specific enumerations. In addition, the principle of non-discrimination is not simply negative right as something to avoid, but also a positive right (Rodriguez-Pinzon & Martin, 2003). That is, duty-bearers have the responsibility to provide special measures for disadvantaged or vulnerable groups, such as preferential treatment or affirmative action.

Older adults have the same right to life as everyone else, regardless of their infirmity, proximity to death, disability, or sickness (Articles 3 and 5). These articles denote that older adults are entitled to self-determination (liberty) in decisions that affect their health and well-being, particularly concerning their medical care and end-of-life preferences. In particular, care and treatment of older adults is prohibited from being cruel or degrading, especially in cases of institutional care. This includes being free from exploitation, abuse, and neglect.

Several of the UDHR provisions have special relevance to older adults. Older adults' right to privacy and right to be free from arbitrary interference (Article 12) apply to their health and personal records, their right to informed consent regarding their medical care. This is also connected to older adults' right to remain in their home as long as possible through supportive aging-in-place policies (UN, 2011). Older adults' right to a family and family caregivers is contained in Article 16, which recognizes and supports the family as the fundamental social unit, and the level at which most social welfare is provided and received. Article 21 is the right to participate in government, which supports the incorporation of the accumulated wisdom and experience of older adults into the governance and maintenance of communities. This also means that older adults have the right to participate in the design and development of policies, programs, and services. Article 22 is the right to social security, which is centered on the right to social protection policies such as non-contributory old-age benefits that guarantee a sufficient minimum income, and related social insurance policies such as retirement, unemployment, or sickness. Older adults have the right to work under Article 23. The only explicit reference to older adults is in Article 25, the right to an adequate standard of living, which includes the right to security in old age. Older adults have the right to education and lifelong learning under Article 26.

International Convention on Civil and Political Rights (ICCPR)

Civil and political rights are important to older adults, despite their being typically associated with economic, social, and cultural rights (UN, 2011). The ICCPR contains the right to self-determination (Article 1) and nondiscrimination (Article 2 and 26) which are fundamental to the rights of older adults, as they are to the principles of rights-based practice (UN, 1966a). Self-determination relates to maintaining dignity and control even as an older adult becomes more dependent, and nondiscrimination is essential to older adults facing ageism. Article 26 reinforces the principle of nondiscrimination (although age is not listed as a ground for prohibiting discrimination) and of equal protection. Article 7, in the right to be free from cruel and degrading treatment and to informed consent, protects older adults from inadequate standards of care in programs, particularly institutions, and to informed consent regarding medical and scientific research. Procedural rights (Article 14), which include equality in courts and tribunals, can be applied to protect older adults against forced retirement or termination of health and social benefits. Articles 18, 19, 21, and 25 include the rights of freedom of expression, assembly, association, and to take part in the affairs of one's own country; these guarantee older adults the principle of participation (Fredvang & Biggs, 2012).

International Covenant on Economic, Social and Cultural Rights (ICESCR)

The ICESCR is the treaty most often linked to the human rights of older adults, and is monitored by the Committee on Economic, Social and Cultural Rights (CESCR) (UN, 1966b). CESCR issued General Comment 6 in 1995 interpreting the ICESCR in the context of older adults. Other General Comments by CESCR that address older adults include No. 14 in 2000 on the right to health, No. 19 in 2008 on the right to social security, and No. 20 in 2009 on nondiscrimination. CESCR frames the state as the primary duty-bearer for the rights of older adults. The economic, social, and cultural rights of older adults are indivisible and interconnected; for example, violations of the right to food, housing, or working conditions will result in violations of the right to health (Huenchuan & Rodriguez-Pinero, 2011; Rodriguez-Pinzon & Martin, 2003; UN, 2011).

Age is among the prohibited grounds of discrimination, and older adults are defined as people 60 years and older. Prohibition against ageism was not included in the UDHR or ICESCR, as the demographic trend toward older adults was not yet visible and the aging of the population had not become a global priority. This is an important example of how human rights are not static but are dynamic, and evolve in concert with changes in human society. Article 3 affirms gender equality; nondiscrimination is particularly relevant to older women vulnerable to economic insecurity due to primary care-taking responsibilities.

Article 11 of the ICESCR contains the rights of older adults to an adequate standard of living, which encompasses the right to food – including vitamins and nutrients, water, shelter, clothing, and health care. This means that old age requires special protection, and states are obligated to provide food, housing, and specialized care through income, family, community, and self-help means governed by national policies and programs. Older adults' right to physical and mental health is identified in Article 12, and includes the right to preventative, environmental, curative, and rehabilitative treatments, and spans both physical and psychological health. Older adults have the right to choose to remain at home, as stated in Article 10.

Older adults' rights to education and culture are contained in Articles 13–15. The human right to education, which cannot be abridged by age, means that older adults have the right to lifelong learning and to pass on their accumulated knowledge and wisdom to younger generations. The rights of older adults to culture encompasses access to cultural institutions and measures to promote their sense of identity and belonging in the community in order to integrate, not segregate, older adults into society.

Older adults' right to work is protected in Articles 6–8. The right to work includes protection against age discrimination during hiring, evaluations, working conditions, and retirement. The right to social security in Article 9 is an entitlement that states must guarantee, essential for older adults unable to find or maintain employment due to old age, disability, or low wage to meet their basic needs. The right to social security may be the most explicit right of older adults, identified in the UDHR, CERD, CEDAW, and CRC.

Convention on the Elimination of All Forms of Discrimination against Women (CEDAW)

The 1979 CEDAW does not reference older adults; however gender equality is understood to be a human right throughout life (UN, 1979). CEDAW affirms equal gender rights to social security (Fredvang & Biggs, 2012). In 2010 the Committee on the Elimination of Discrimination against Women published General Recommendation No. 27 (GR 27) pertaining to the rights of older women. GR 27 clarified that all the rights contained in CEDAW apply to women of all ages and that it prohibits ageism. It also clarified the need to eliminate negative stereotypes and social and cultural patterns, and emphasized the participation of older women in all spheres of society. Discrimination in marriage and inheritance laws and practices should be repealed to afford older women access to housing, property, and land (UN, 2011). GR 27 addresses civil and political rights by discussing states' obligations to protect older women from physical, sexual, psychological, verbal, and economic abuse, to combat violence against older women, and to train law enforcement and justice professionals on the rights of older women (Huenchuan & Rodriguez-Pinero, 2011). GR 27 explains that states have the responsibility to protect older women from violence, including harm that results from traditional beliefs or practices. GR 27 also specifies the rights of older women to include the access to non-contributory old-age benefits, to stay at home as long as possible and to live independently, and to caregiver support.

Other international and regional documents

Additional human rights conventions apply to the rights of older adults. The 1984 Convention against Torture and Other Cruel, Inhuman or Degrading Treatment or Punishment has been interpreted to apply to institutional care for older adults, requiring states to prevent mistreatment (UN, 2011). Article 7 of the 1990 International Convention on the Protection of the Rights of All Migrant Workers and Members of their Families explicitly identifies age as a form of discrimination (Fredvang & Biggs, 2012; UN, 1990).

The 2006 Convention on the Rights of Persons with Disabilities (CRPD) also prohibits discrimination on the basis of age and calls for age-appropriate accommodations and age-sensitive assistance for older adults with disabilities to ensure access to their rights to health care, social protection, and anti-poverty programs (UN, 2006). This includes services required specifically due to disability that might minimize or prevent disability among older adults. The CRPD also links independent living, personal mobility, and habitation as well as access to justice and freedom from exploitation to older adults.

Regional human rights systems have also articulated the human rights of older adults (Huenchuan & Rodriguez-Pinero, 2011; Kollapan, 2008; Rodriguez-Pinzon & Martin, 2003; Tang & Lee, 2006). The European Social Charter protects older adults' rights to participation, social protection, health care, and housing, in order to remain full members of society for as long as possible. The EU's Charter of Fundamental Rights also respects the rights of older adults to dignity, independence, and nondiscrimination. The Inter-American Commission for Human Rights, in revisions to the 1988 Protocol of San Salvador, protects the rights of older adults and refers to them as an especially vulnerable population requiring prioritized protections. The Andean Charter prohibits discrimination on the basis of age. The African Charter on Human and People's Rights of 1986 acknowledges the need for special measures of protection for older adults and affirms the value of family in protecting and caring for older adults, as does the African Youth Charter and the Protocol to the African Charter on the Rights of Women in Africa.

Growing international consensus

International consensus of the need for a specific convention on the rights of older adults is growing (Huenchuan & Rodriguez-Pinero, 2011; Rodriguez-Pinzon & Martin, 2003; Tang & Lee, 2006). Beginning in 1973, the UN General Assembly called for the protection of the rights of older persons. In 1982, the UN held the first World Assembly on Ageing in Vienna, resulting in the International Plan of Action on Aging (the Vienna Plan), the first step towards global recognition of older adults' human rights (Tang & Lee, 2006). Recommendations included prioritizing social inclusion – especially for rural and older women – community-based and home-based care, combating stereotypes, and affirming the value and dignity of older adults.

In 1991 the UN adopted Principles for Older Persons, which included inter-dependence (including basic needs, income, and education), participation, care (regardless of living at home or institutionalized), and self-fulfillment through access to cultural and educational resources, and dignity in the freedom from abuse and discrimination. These principles have yet to be translated into specific standards in a comprehensive manner.

Madrid International Plan of Action on Ageing (MIPAA)

The UN declared 1999 the International Year of Older Persons and in 2002 held the Second World Assembly on Ageing in Madrid, resulting in the Madrid International Plan of Action on Ageing (MIPAA). MIPAA promoted the rights of older adults in global agendas by outlining three priority directions for action: development, health, and enabling and supportive environments (UN, 2011). The first priority recognized the need to ensure the economic stability and social protection of older adults from vulnerability, especially in times of emergency, disaster, and conflict. Proposals included social security, aging-friendly employment opportunities, and a minimum income for older adults. The second priority of advancing older adults' health and well-being included policy prescriptions for reducing health risks and disease, comprehensive mental health care services including prevention, and eliminating inequalities in health care. The third priority of enabling and supportive environments included protecting older adults from abuse and neglect with affordable, accessible, and culturally competent social services.

MIPAA accelerated global awareness of older adults' rights and calls for a convention intensified (Huenchuan & Rodriguez-Pinero, 2011). The 2007 Brasilia Declaration called for a Special Rapporteur on Ageing to examine the rights of older adults and promote good practices. In 2011 the UN Secretary-General noted that despite MIPAA's positive developments, gaps remain for more specific and explicit protections. Several NGOs, such as Help Age International, the International Federation on Ageing, and the Council on Ageing, have called for a Convention on the Rights of Older Persons as a new international human rights instrument that would explicitly protect the rights of older adults.

Proposals for a Convention on the Rights of Older Persons (CROP)

A CROP would create the legal framework and support to promote and protect the rights of older adults in the world's increasingly aging communities (Huenchuan & Rodriguez-Pinero, 2011). The new convention would contain entitlement rights, protection mechanisms, and imperatives for states to utilize resources to realize older adults' rights. A CROP would prohibit all forms of discrimination and violence against older adults, outline their rights to comprehensive and accessible health care, long-term care, medication, and programs to promote aging-in-place and reduce dependency. A CROP would have a committee monitoring state parties' implementation, interpret Convention provisions with General Comments, and receive complaints from individuals or organizations about violations of the rights of older adults (Tang & Lee, 2006). States and NGOs could submit reports assessing the status of older adults.

Supporters of a CROP, including many states from the Global South and NGOs, argue that extant human rights protections are insufficient for older adults, who experience specific human rights violations due to their age, such as ageism (Fredvang & Biggs, 2012; Huenchuan & Rodriguez-Pinero, 2011). Their own convention will raise awareness and influence perceptions and behavior to combat ageism and promote the dignity of older adults. A CROP would acknowledge the discrimination faced by older adults in work, health care, and housing. A new convention would be comprehensive, replacing the disparate existing standards. Proponents see benefit for women and children in the CEDAW and CRC, which can be a model for a CROP (Tang & Lee, 2006). A CROP could prompt states to develop policies and programs by clarifying their obligations toward older adults. The CROP could contribute to a paradigm shift by changing public perception, building public will, transforming the traditional view of older adults into rights–holders, from objects of need to genuine subjects of rights. A CROP could combat negative stereotypes, prejudiced attitudes, and discriminatory practices against older adults by increasing older adults' visibility. In addition to a legal impact, a CROP could also highlight the positive and productive contributions that older adults make to younger generations and to society. A CROP would acknowledge older adults' vulnerability and unique challenges in an integrative framework and ensure that they are included in global agendas. International protections of the rights of older adults would be strengthened by the CROP's supervisory mechanisms and subject area experts monitoring implementation by state parties.

However, some states have raised objections to a CROP; the U.S., EU, Norway, Russia, New Zealand, and China contend that separate human rights protections are redundant and fragment the universalism of all rights. Instead of a new convention that would lack sufficient enforcement, existing protections should be strengthened and made enforceable. Current treaties are overwhelmed and plagued by a lack of accountability or sanctions. In the past, states have used the rhetoric of embracing new agreements in order to give the superficial appearance of allegiance to human rights values rather than commit to meaningful social change (Fredvang & Biggs, 2012). These states claim that energy on behalf of a CROP would be better spent ensuring that governments and civil society protect the rights of older adults on the ground by advocating for adequate policy and program provisions. Opponents argue that highlighting the differences between older adults and other adults contributes to their stigmatization and marginalization.

Case study of rights-based approaches with older adults

HelpAge International (HAI)

HelpAge International (HAI) defines itself as a global movement for the rights of older people (www.helpage.org). Founded in 1983 by NGOs in Canada, Colombia, Kenya, India, and the U.K., HAI was created to lobby for the rights of older refugees fleeing conflict in East Africa who were not being served by traditional agencies due to their age. Early programs focused on eye care and community-based services. In 1988 these initial national and regional NGOs merged into a global network that continues to grow, consisting of over 100 allied organizations in 65 countries. HAI is guided by the belief of the value of older adults' contribution to society. Their mission is to promote the rights of older people to live dignified, secure, active, and healthy lives free of discrimination and poverty. HAI embodies participation by placing older adults at the center of their program planning and evaluation. HAI provides services, partners with local organizations, evaluates their programs, and advocates for policymakers to engage with older adults and protect their rights. HAI engages in participatory research with older adults, leads international campaigns, and makes policy recommendations for serving older adults.

HAI works with local partners around the world to promote older adults' rights to physical security, social services, and health care. They provide partnering organizations with technical assistance in the form of fundraising support, skills transfer, and resources to build capacity of the global movement. HAI also conducts trainings and workshops on helping older adults in emergencies, developing pension programs, working with the media, and older citizens' monitoring. HAI issues press releases, newsletters, and videos of older adults to promote awareness and sensitivity of the special vulnerability of older adults.

HAI is funded by grants from governmental, UN, and development organizations. Most of its nearly $40 million (USD) annual budget is spent in Africa and Asia on humanitarian relief in emergencies, health care, secure incomes, and fighting age discrimination. Expenditures include small grants to local and regional partners in every region across the world. HAI holds itself accountable to older adults through external evaluations, regular program reviews, and sharing their strategic planning. HAI consults with the UN and WHO and helped to shape the Madrid Plan.

As an NGO that focuses on the specific vulnerabilities and needs of older adults, HAI promotes their inclusion in humanitarian relief. HAI facilitates older adults' participation in aid efforts and coordinates task forces to address the needs of older adults. HAI helps older adults to cope with climate change and collaborates with disaster risk reduction programs to reduce the vulnerability of older adults to natural disasters. HAI works with health care providers to meet the health needs of global aging, including dementia and cancer. Special effort is made to address the health of older adults with HIV/AIDS and caregivers of HIV/AIDS orphans. HAI also works to enable secure incomes for older adults, and focuses on developing social protection programs to reduce poverty. Pensions and access to decent work are the foremost strategies to ensuring a regular and predictable income for older adults.

Along with many human rights advocates, HAI is concerned that existing human rights protections are insufficient for protecting the rights of older adults. HAI's advocacy is centered on building support for a Convention on the Rights of Older People and for older adults to claim their rights in local contexts. HAI's main advocacy campaign is called Age Demands Action. The Age Demands Action campaign utilizes marches, debates, and petitions to advocate at multiple levels for the Convention on the Rights of Older People. Beginning in 2007 with 27 countries, the campaign has expanded to 65 countries in 2014 and has engaged an estimated 62,000 campaigners. During this time, over 20 countries have developed social policies on older adults, 17 extended social protection for older adults, 11 improved health services for older adults, seven created national committees of older people, and HAI consulted with four states to develop policies for older adults. In addition to promoting the Convention on the Rights of Older Persons, HAI campaigns have challenged age discrimination and stereotypes of older adults as nonproductive and drains upon household resources, and have led to improved health services, access to public transportation, and special discounts.

A major advocacy tool that HAI developed is the Global AgeWatch Index. The Global AgeWatch Index ranks countries on assessments of older adults' well-being in terms of income, health, employment, education and enabling environments. This index is a valuable new tool for stimulating debate, comparative studies, and raising awareness of older adults' well-being in different countries.

HAI has had a significant impact upon raising awareness of aging issues, particularly in the Global South among countries undergoing rapid demographic transitions. HAI has worked with 1.5 million vulnerable older adults through 3,000 associations. An estimated 1.35 million older adults are eligible for pensions where HAI has advocated reforms, and they have helped 250,000 older adults access health care. HAI recently conducted major relief operations in the Philippines following Typhoon Haiyan. HAI has created older adults citizens' monitoring groups for older people to learn about and advocate for their rights. HAI has facilitated older adults speaking at the WHO NGO Forum on Ageing and was recognized in 2012 with the world's largest humanitarian prize.

Rights-based approaches to social work practice with older adults

Global aging presents opportunities and responsibilities for social workers to build upon their strengths of working with older adults to implement rights-based approaches (Huenchuan & Rodriguez-Pinero, 2011; Mukherjee, 2009; Tang & Lee, 2006). Rights-based social work practice should promote healthy and active aging. The IFSW Statement on Aging calls for more gerontological social workers that can protect older adults against elder abuse and neglect, promote their economic and social stability, ensure the accessibility and delivery of quality health care, and prevent isolation and depression. A rights-based approach to older adults is consistent with gerontological practice that emphasizes individuals' strengths and the centrality of their family and community relationships.

Rights-based approaches with older adults will promote their human dignity (Huenchuan & Rodriguez-Pinero, 2011). This involves shifting the paradigm away from viewing older adults as needy, helpless dependents whose contributions are behind them, with nothing of value left to offer society. Instead older adults are to be viewed as empowered agents, deserving of as much rights as others at any life stage, who have the right to be fully integrated into every aspect of society, as fully realized subjects. Rights-based approaches should promote positive and realistic images of older adults and aging to encourage appreciation of older adults.

Human dignity for older adults requires their autonomy and self-determination. This means that practitioners should respect the rights of older adults to make their own informed decisions about their use of social, legal, and medical services and care, including decisions about end-of-life care. This applies to where older adults are in long-term home and institutional care. However the principle of dignity for older adults also builds upon social work approaches to promote community care and active aging (Tang & Lee, 2006). Social workers should enable older adults to remain physically, politically, socially, and economically active as long as possible, for as long as they are able and want to remain living independently, which benefits themselves as well as communities.

Dignity also pertains to social work practice that protects the personal integrity of older adults, by preventing exploitation, abuse, mistreatment, and neglect. This includes promoting the right to a dignified death. Older adults with terminal conditions or who are dying should have access to palliative care to promote a dignified and painless death. Care should not be restricted at the end of life due to lack of ability to pay. Rights-based approaches include advance directives that incorporate the right of older adults to make those decisions and to have their wishes respected even when they can't communicate them.

The principle of nondiscrimination in rights-based approaches with older adults means recognizing that the rights of older adults are uniquely vulnerable and deserving of special attention and protection, and specifically preventing and punishing age-based discrimination. Policies and programs for older adults should be both specific and mainstream; age-friendly approaches should be specifically tailored for older adults and mainstreamed across existing policies.

Practice priorities include preventing and rectifying ageism that contributes to social isolation and marginalization of older adults, by fostering aging-in-place and community integration (Huenchuan & Rodriguez-Pinero, 2011). Social work practice with older adults recognizes that all people regardless of age have rights and an active role to play in contributing to society. This means attending to the structural disadvantages affecting older adults (Rodriguez-Pinzon & Martin, 2003). Indigenous, rural, and migrant older adults are subgroups of older adults who are at greater vulnerability and require special attention.

Nondiscrimination means that services should be made accessible to older adults who choose to live at home (Rodriguez-Pinzon & Martin, 2003). Rights-based practice with older adults means fostering enabling and supportive environments. Social work practice should facilitate aging-in-place (Huenchuan & Rodriguez-Pinero,

2011). Social workers can support families and promote aging-in-place through providing transportation, food delivery, nursing care, and medical visits. Caregiver relief also supports the cultural value and practice of older adults being cared for by their families. Supporting older adults in their home as long as possible may entail restoring, developing, improving, or adapting the residence.

Older adults cannot be denied access to services and programs available to the rest of the population. For example, in order to protect older adults' right to work, technical, professional, and higher education should be made accessible to older adults, in particular older women and older adults with disabilities. Rights-based approaches must incorporate nondiscrimination in other areas, such as the right to housing of older adults. Practitioners should work to ensure affordability such as with housing subsidies and protection against forced eviction and unreasonable rent increases. Older adults must be guaranteed adequate and habitable housing, which includes protection from cold and heat, and access to safe drinking water, energy, heat, light, and sanitation. Practitioners must also attend to the geographical and cultural accessibility of housing for older adults, as in nearby employment and educational sites, and allowing for cultural expression and technological advances.

Rights-based approaches with older adults also promote their full participation in society. Older adults' right to participation pertains to political, cultural, and social dimensions. Incorporating older adults' right to participation means attending to the element of process in social work practice. Social workers should ensure the participation of older adults in the development of health care services, including long-term care. Above all, practitioners must include the participation of older adults in decision making and planning processes at all levels. This would enable their voices to affect decisions impinging their welfare in all levels of government and administration and in neighborhoods and community-based organizations. Social work practice can realize older adults' right to participation by strengthening their access to and quality of social capital, increasing the role of civil society, and encouraging their involvement in voluntary associations and organizations. Social workers should work to organize older adults to work for older adults' rights, and to empower their social networks.

Principles of transparency and accountability are core aspects of social work practice with older adults. To promote a conducive environment for rights-based approaches, social workers should advocate for policies that move beyond a social welfare orientation towards older adults. Priorities include transparent and accountable programs and policies that guarantee older adults an adequate standard of living, health care, education, housing, work, and social security. Social workers must not neglect the rights of isolated older adults in long-term care institutions or those in detention.

Rights-based approaches should include advocacy that educates the general public about the rights of older adults. Age-friendly perspectives should be incorporated into the design and delivery of programs and services to promote the active and independent living of older adults. Social workers can engage in policy practice within states to facilitate the promotion and adoption of social protection policies.

Social workers should also focus on ensuring that older adults' programs and policies are sufficiently funded, through grant writing, fundraising, or social development policies (Midgley, 2014).

Social workers should join international efforts in advocating for a Convention on the Rights of Older Persons. Social workers should also contribute to building international consortiums that foster support for international frameworks supporting the rights of older adults (Mukherjee, 2009). Advancing older adults' rights depends on the international mobilization of older adults, social workers, and civil society.

Rights-based social work practice should promote universal access to health care for older adults and ensure their equal access to health care facilities and services, food, and nutrition. Practitioners should work to promote older adults' right to health, including periodic check-ups, treatment for the chronically and terminally ill, and free emergency health care. Social workers should work to prohibit experimentation and treatment of older adults without their informed consent, and prevent interference with older adults' decisions regarding their health care.

Rights-based approaches with older adults also involve education. Social workers should develop informal, community-based, and recreation-oriented programs that foster older adults' self-reliance and community responsibility. Practitioners must ensure older adults' access to continuing education, training and re-training programs, and vocational guidance and placement services. Older-adult education programs should be implemented in community centers where younger people have access to their experiences and insights. Intergenerational communication enriches society and strengthens solidarity. Social workers should advocate for financial assistance that ensures older adults' access to education programs.

Rights-based approaches with older adults require more research to document and publicize patterns of violations of their rights and to strengthen social work practice in the field of gerontology. Aging concepts and information on the rights of older adults should be incorporated into all levels of social work education.

Social work practice with older adults must also support policies that protect their right to an adequate standard of living through non-contributory old-age benefits, social pensions, and old-age insurance programs that guarantee older adults and their families a minimum income. Such programs that protect older adults from poverty are often cost-effective for states in the Global South, at less than 1% of GDP, where they are becoming more widespread. Social workers should also advocate for policies that protect older adults' right to work through flexible retirement ages and programs that reward, not penalize, older workers for their experience, perhaps through lateral promotions rather than demotions. Older workers should also be educated about retirement and vocational training programs. Social workers should work for the public recognition of the productivity and contributions of older adults.

For further reading on rights-based approaches with older adults

AARP

U.S. nonprofit with over 37 million members promoting dignity of older adults and lobbying for economic security, health and long-term care, livable communities, consumer protection, and participation.
www.aarp.org/ and www.aarpinternational.org/

Global Action on Aging

A nonprofit in New York that consults with the UN promoting awareness of older adults needs and potential.
http://globalaging.blogspot.com/

Global Alliance for the Rights of Older People

Alliance working to strengthen the rights and voice of older adults globally.
www.rightsofolderpeople.org/

International Association of Gerontology and Geriatrics

Promoting research and training in gerontological research to enhance older adults' well-being.
www.iagg.info/

International Association of Homes and Services for the Ageing

A global network of experts in services, housing, research, and technology for older adults.
www./iahsa.net/

International Federation on Ageing

Network of NGOs, corporations, academics, and governments working for positive change for older adults.
www.ifa-fiv.org/

International Network for the Prevention of Elder Abuse

Promoting advocacy, education, and research protecting the rights of older adults through global dissemination.
www.inpea.net/

UN Open-ended Working Group on Ageing

Reviews international framework of rights of older adults to identify gaps.
http://social.un.org/ageing-working-group/

World Health Organization Department of Ageing and Life Course

WHO agency promoting rights of older adults as a global priority.
www.who.int/ageing/en/

References

Fredvang, M., & Biggs, S. (2012). *The rights of older persons: Protection and gaps under human rights law.* Social Policy Working Paper no. 16. Centre for Public Policy & Brotherhood of St. Laurence. Melbourne: University of Melbourne. Retrieved from: http://social.un.org/ageing-working-group/documents/fourth/Rightsofolderpersons.pdf

Giunta, N. (2010). Productive aging and social development. In J. Midgely & A. Conley (Eds.), *Social work and social development: Theories and skills for developmental social work* (pp. 55–70). New York: Oxford University Press.

Guseilo, J., Curl, A., & Hokenstad, M. (2004). Policies and programs in aging: International initiatives. In M. Hokenstand & J. Midgley (Eds.), *Lessons from abroad: Adapting international social welfare innovations* (pp. 13–30). Washington, DC: NASW Press.

Hokenstad, T., & Choi, M. (2012). Global aging. In L. Healy & R. Link (Eds.), *Handbook of international social work: Human rights, development, and the global profession* (pp. 137–141). Oxford: Oxford University Press.

Hokenstad, T., & Roberts, A. (2012). Older persons and social work: A global perspective. In K. Lyons, T. Hokenstad, M. Pawar, N. Huegler, & N. Hall (Eds.), *The SAGE handbook of international social work* (pp. 372–387). Thousand Oaks, CA: Sage.

Huenchuan, S., & Rodriguez-Pinero, L. (2011). *Ageing and the protection of human rights: Current situation and outlook.* United Nations. Santiago, Chile: Economic Commission for Latin America and the Caribbean. Retrieved from: http://social.un.org/ageing-working-group/documents/ECLAC_Ageing and the protection of human rights_current situation and outlook_Project document.pdf

International Labour Organization (ILO). (2014). *World Social Protection Report 2014/15: Building economic recovery, inclusive development and social justice.* Geneva: Author. Retrieved from: www.ilo.org/wcmsp5/groups/public/—-dgreports/—-dcomm/documents/publication/wcms_245201.pdf

Kollapan, J. (2008). *The rights of older people – African perspectives.* South Africa Human Rights Commission. New York: Global Action on Aging. Retrieved from: www.globalaging.org/elderrights/world/2008/africa.pdf

Midgley, J. (2014). *Social development: Theory and practice.* Los Angeles: Sage.

Mukherjee, D. (2009). Global aging and international social work practice: A developing country perspective. *Journal of Global Social Work Practice, 2*(1).

Rodriguez-Pinzon, D., & Martin, C. (2003). The international human rights status of elderly persons. *American University International Law Review, 18*(4), 915–1008.

Tang, K., & Lee, J. (2006). Global social justice for older people: The case for an international convention on the rights of older people. *British Journal of Social Work, 36*(7), 1135–1150.

United Nations (UN). (1948, December 10). Universal Declaration of Human Rights. UN General Assembly. Retrieved from: www.un.org/Overview/rights.htm

United Nations (UN). (1966a). *International Covenant on Civil and Political Rights.* New York: Author. Retrieved from: www.ohchr.org/en/professionalinterest/pages/ccpr.aspx

United Nations (UN). (1966b). *International Covenant on Economic, Social and Cultural Rights.* New York: Author. Retrieved from: www.ohchr.org/EN/ProfessionalInterest/Pages/CESCR.aspx

United Nations (UN). (1979). *Convention on the Elimination of All Forms of Discrimination Against Women.* New York: Author. Retrieved from: www.un.org/womenwatch/daw/cedaw/text/econvention.htm

United Nations (UN). (1989). *General Comment No. 18: Non-discrimination.* New York: UN Human Rights Committee. Retrieved from: http://tbinternet.ohchr.org/_layouts/treatybodyexternal/Download.aspx?symbolno=INT%2fCCPR%2fGEC%2f6622&Lang=en

United Nations (UN). (1990). *International Convention on the Protection for the Rights of All Migrant Workers and Members of Their Families*. New York: Author. Retrieved from: www2. ohchr.org/english/bodies/cmw/cmw.htm

United Nations (UN). (2006). *Convention on the Rights of Persons with Disabilities*. New York: Author. Retrieved from: www.un.org/disabilities/convention/conventionfull.shtml

United Nations (UN). (2010). *General Recommendation No. 27 on Older Women and Protection of Their Human Rights*. New York: Committee on the Elimination of Discrimination Against Women. Retrieved from: www2.ohchr.org/english/bodies/cedaw/docs/CEDAW-C-2010-47-GC1.pdf

United Nations (UN). (2011). *Human rights of older persons: References from some international human rights treaties and the MIPAA*. Open-ended working group on ageing for the purpose of strengthening the protection of the human rights of older persons. New York: UN Programme on Ageing, Division for Social Policy and Development, UN Department of Economic and Social Affairs. Retrieved from: http://social.un.org/ageing-working-group/documents/Table HR & MIPAA – April 2011.pdf

Wong, E. (2013, July 2). A Chinese virtue in now the law. *New York Times*. Retrieved from: www.nytimes.com/2013/07/03/world/asia/filial-piety-once-a-virtue-in-china-is-now-the-law.html?_r=0

6

HUMAN RIGHTS-BASED APPROACHES TO HEALTH

Health is fundamental to well-being and thus a human right. The tragedy of deaths due to preventable causes and the specter of global epidemics underscore the importance of human health and access to health care. The 2014 Ebola outbreak in West Africa demonstrates the fragility and interconnectedness of global health. Disease, sickness, and ill health result in lost years of life and productivity. One hundred fifty million people suffer financial catastrophe each year due to health-related costs (WHO, 2013). One hundred million people sink into poverty due to health-related costs. The UN estimates that over 25 million people have died in the AIDS epidemic in the last 25 years. Currently 33 million people are living with AIDS; a destructive, major health pandemic catastrophe with grave implications for public health, human rights, and social work. Unsafe water and poor sanitation and hygiene contribute to diarrhea that caused 2.7% of global deaths in 2002, or 1.5 million people (Fewtrell, Pruss-Ustun, Bos, Gore & Bartram, 2007). These issues have become a global priority, as evidenced by the Millennium Development Goals targets for reducing preventable diseases, improving maternal health, and increasing access to clean water and sanitation.

Traditional approaches to health

Social work approaches to health have been heavily influenced by the fields of medicine and public health. At least since the infamous 1915 speech by Abraham Flexner and subsequent publication of Mary Richmond's *Social Diagnosis* (1917), social work has looked to medicine as a model for professional practice. This conscious adoption of the medical model has had a dramatic impact on the profession, and its influence continues today. The medical model's influence upon social work has been criticized for its deficit-based approach that inherently pathologizes the issue that the practitioner is focused on. The diagnosis-then-treatment model of intervention has been a defining focus of social work in the U.S.

Unfortunately, human rights violations are committed in the name of medical and health interventions (Amon, 2010). One need not go as far back as the Nazi human experiments or the American syphilis study to find examples. Disadvantaged populations, such as racial, ethnic, and religious minorities, transgender people, and drug-users, are frequently at risk for substandard care or denials of medical treatment. Forcible sterilizations, denials of life-saving abortions, unnecessary genital examinations of sexual minorities, and denial of treatment of stigmatized populations are but a few of the violations of the right to health faced by people around the world. Health professionals are sometimes complicit in torture, and inhumane and degrading treatment through the denial of medical care (PHR, 2008).

There has been a growth of social work practice roles in various health care settings, such as in emergency rooms and hospice care. Medical social work includes specialty practice in oncology and public health. Social work in health is characterized by practice in interdisciplinary teams with allied health and medical professionals. Recent exciting developments in the field of health that complement rights-based approaches include understanding the social determinants of health, a focus on reducing health disparities, and the emergence of global public health. Joint MSW and MPH programs are becoming more common with the rise of attention to global health from the nonprofit and charitable sector.

To move beyond the medical model, health should be framed positively. Instead of conceptualizing of health as the absence of disease, it should be reframed as a form of wellness (Nadkarni & Vikram, 2009). The medical model also tends to be individualistic, and has contributed to an individualistic emphasis within social work. Re-conceptualizing health means moving beyond biological and technological interventions and attending to social conditions that affect the promotion, protection, and maintenance of health.

The human right to health

There is widespread consensus in the human rights community that the right to health means that states are responsible for creating and maintaining conditions for all people to be as healthy as possible (UN, 2008; WHO, 2013; Zuniga, Marks & Gostin, 2013). Although human rights related to health have been typically viewed as part of economic, social, and cultural rights, they are indivisible and interconnected with all other rights. Health is linked to many extant human rights; victims of violations by violence, torture, and forced labor experience health consequences. Health policies and services can violate human rights. The right to health includes both negative and positive rights, and is a good example of the false dichotomy. The human right to health is both a singular right in and of itself, and a right fundamentally related to other rights which have a direct bearing on people's health. The right to health is linked to the right to certain social and environmental conditions that influence people's health, such as the rights to food and nutrition, water and sanitation, housing, and health-related information and technology.

The treaty body with the most overview on the right to health is the Committee on Economic, Social and Cultural Rights. Other treaty bodies such as the Committee on the Elimination of Racial Discrimination, the Committee on the Elimination of Discrimination against Women, and the Committee on the Rights of the Child also consider matters related to the right to health. The Committee against Torture also covers the right to health for people held in detention and institutions, including psychiatric institutions, and for victims recovering from torture and sexual violence.

Definition

Humans have the right to the highest attainable standard of health. The right to health is more than the right to health care, and includes the freedom to control a person's own health (UN, 2008). The right to health is distinguished as distinct from the right to be healthy; genetic and biological differences affect individuals' health. The right to health depends upon the underlying and necessary conditions of health, such as access to and availability of health care, adequate water, food, and housing, safe working conditions, and protection from violence, trauma, and oppression (WHO, 2013). All states are party to at least one human rights agreement addressing health-related rights. States are obligated to the progressive realization of the right to health, and to cooperate in the respecting of the right to health in other state jurisdictions.

Nondiscrimination is a key element of the right to health, as populations subject to discrimination, inequality, and marginalization bear the brunt of disease and poor health outcomes (Claude & Weston, 2006; Hunt, 2006). Discrimination is a core cause of ill health, and nondiscrimination means differential treatment in order to reduce inequalities and disparities (WHO, 2002). People cannot be discriminated against on the basis of health status. Health care systems are heavily influenced by patterns of social privilege, which is so prevalent that all health programs should be considered discriminatory until they can demonstrate nondiscrimination (Mann, 1997).

History

Health was on the agenda of early human rights pioneers; the 1946 WHO constitution predates the 1948 UDHR (Gruskin, Mills & Tarantola, 2007). However, health remained disconnected from human rights discourse through most of the Cold War; the emergence of the HIV/AIDS epidemic and attention to sexual and reproductive health initiated a reconnection. The 1978 Declaration of Alma-Ata reiterated the connection between health and human rights. The Declaration prioritized primary health care and the realization of the highest attainable standard of health. The WHO Global Program on AIDS led by Jonathan Mann highlighted the role of discrimination and stigma in restricting people's access to health care prevention and treatment. International consensus slowly emerged to make health policies and programs accountable to human rights. A series of UN conferences and the World Health Assembly combined the experiences of health workers around the world and formally endorsed the right to health.

World Health Organization (WHO)

The 1946 WHO constitution was the first international declaration of health as a human right and defined health as "a state of complete physical, mental and social well-being and not merely the absence of disease or infirmity" (WHO, 1946, p. 1). The constitution mandated WHO with global leadership on health, and prioritized child development, equitable dissemination of medical research, and state measures to promote health. The WHO has embraced a rights-based approach to health and seeks to build capacity of states and NGOs to implement the right to health (Nadkarni & Vikram, 2009; WHO, 2013). The 2005 WHO Commission on the Social Determinants of Health linked health to human rights by identifying the structural patterns of hierarchal privilege, power, and access to resources as associated with health disparities and inequalities of care (WHO, 2008). This Commission highlighted the right to participate in health care policy debates and program design. The WHO seeks to develop rights-based health indicators, monitor health policies, conduct trainings on health and human rights, and attend to special populations such as indigenous people's health and human rights. The WHO also establishes health standards and treaties, such as the 1981 International Code of Marketing of Breast Milk Substitutes and the 2003 Framework Convention on Tobacco Control.

Universal Declaration of Human Rights (UDHR)

The UDHR identifies the right to health as a fundamental right of every human being in Article 25, and specifically protects the right to maternity care (UN, 1948). The universality of the UDHR demonstrates that all human rights are necessary for health.

International Covenant on Civil and Political Rights (ICCPR)

The ICCPR identifies the right to freedoms necessary for health (UN, 1966a). Article 7 prohibits torture and cruel, inhuman, or degrading treatment or punishment, and contains the principle of informed consent in the freedom from medical or scientific experimentation without consent. Articles 12 and 17 mandate the right to privacy, which relates to confidentiality and the right to have one's medical information and records kept private. Article 19 contains the right to information, which is relevant to knowledge about health-related interventions necessary to make informed decisions about care; this is a core principle of evidence-based care (Gambrill, 2006).

International Covenant on Economic, Social and Cultural Rights (ICESCR)

The ICESCR proclaims the human right to the highest attainable standard of physical and mental health (Article 12) (UN, 1966b). The right to health depends upon the right to basic resources, such as the right to food, nutrition, water, sanitation, housing, work, education, information, and medical care and necessary social services (Articles 11 and 12) (UN, 2000). Mothers are entitled to special protections before and after childbirth (Article 10), which includes paid leave or leave with adequate social security benefits for working mothers. Specific building blocks to realizing the right to health include maternal and child health, sanitation, disease prevention and control, and equal access to health care (Article 12).

The right to health in the ICESCR also includes the right to health-related education such as basic knowledge of child health and nutrition, the advantages of breastfeeding, hygiene and environmental sanitation, and the prevention of accidents (Article 14). The right to the benefits of scientific progress, medical research and technology is included in Article 15.

General Comment 14 (GC 14)

In 2000 the Committee on Economic, Social, and Cultural Rights released GC 14 on the right to health. GC 14 emphasizes that the right to health is related to the social determinants of health, and broadens the right to health beyond the right to health care to the right to underlying conditions that promote health (Hunt, 2007; UN, 2000; WHO, 2013). GC 14 defines the minimum essential of the right to health, which includes essential primary health care, essential drugs, minimum essential and nutritious food, safe and potable water, shelter, housing and sanitation. GC 14 defines health equity as nondiscrimination in health care, facilities, personnel, and goods and services, including for those without sufficient means or health insurance. The principle of nondiscrimination in the right to health prioritizes people's health over their social status. It also means reducing and eliminating health disparities and attending to the underlying conditions which cause disparities. GC 14 identifies four elements of the right to health: availability of health care facilities, programs, personnel, and services; accessibility for all without discrimination, including affordability; acceptability of care relative to culture, gender, and age; and good quality and medically appropriate care.

GC 14 elaborates the three obligations of states as the duty to respect, protect, and fulfill the right to health. Respecting the right to health means non-interference, such as preventing unsafe medication, health misinformation, privacy violations, and denials of health care. Protecting the right to health means preventing the infringement of people's health by third-party, non-state actors, such as through regulation of the private market and traditional practices. Fulfilling the right to health requires states to make positive contributions, such as implementing policies, budgets, and programs that will enable people to enjoy the right to health. States are obligated to develop national health policies that address public and private sectors, immunization programs, prevention services, nondiscrimination, safe and nutritious food, sanitation and water, public health infrastructure, sexual and reproductive health services and information, training for professionals, and resources for health-related issues such as HIV/AIDS, substance abuse, and domestic violence. Additional state obligations include international cooperation, such as in emergency relief; progressive realization according to available resources; and taking immediate steps towards nondiscrimination and starting the process of progressive realization.

International Convention on the Elimination of All Forms of Racial Discrimination (CERD)

The 1965 CERD contains the right of all racial and ethnic groups, including racial minorities, to public health and medical care (Article 5) (UN, 1965). Discrimination is a key factor in perpetuating health disparities; racism and xenophobia are health detriments and contribute to inequality (Nadkarni & Vikram, 2009; WHO, 2008).

Convention on the Elimination of All Forms of Discrimination against Women (CEDAW)

The 1979 CEDAW incorporates the right to health, and prioritizes gender equality in access to health care services (Article 12) (UN, 1979). CEDAW notes women's right to participate in and access to health care and family planning, especially rural women (Article 14). CEDAW prohibits violence against women and harmful traditional practices against women (Article 11). Reproductive and maternal health is outlined in the right to family planning services, emergency obstetrics, appropriate services for pregnancy, birth, and post-natal, including nutrition and lactation (Article 12). Maternal health care should be free when necessary. States are obligated to provide health care to women in confinement, particularly pregnancy and post-natal maternal health care, and to provide for adequate nutrition during pregnancy and lactation.

Convention on the Rights of the Child (CRC)

The CRC affirms that children have the right to the highest possible standard of health, and that no children should be denied access to health care services (UN, 1989). Children's right to health includes the rights to adequate food and water, access to preventative and primary health care, and freedom from environmental pollution. It states that access to essential medical care for children and pre- and post-natal maternal care are human rights, including information about child health, nutrition, breastfeeding, hygiene, and environmental sanitation and the prevention of accidents. The CRC prioritizes the prevention and reduction of infant and child mortality (Nadkarni & Vikram, 2009). Children have the right to be free from physical, mental, and sexual violence, injury, and abuse, and neglect and exploitation (Article 19). This includes the freedom from traditional practices that cause harm, adverse health consequences, or negative impacts on child and adolescent development (Article 24).

Convention on the Rights of Persons with Disabilities (CRPD)

The 2006 CRPD includes the right to the highest attainable standard of health for persons with disabilities, who are entitled to equal quality health care such as the prevention, identification, and management of disabilities (Article 25) (UN, 2006). The underlying determinants of health are addressed in the CRPD prohibitions against denying health care, food, water, and insurance on the basis of disability. People with disabilities have the right to health care and services in their local communities, in a manner that is geographically equitable. Informed consent is a core health right of people with disabilities, and protection from practices such as institutionalization and sterilization.

Convention on the Rights of Migrant Workers and their Families (CRMW)

The 1990 CRMW recognizes the rights of all migrant workers and their families to health and safe and healthy working conditions regardless of their legal status, documentation, work status, or location (Article 25) (UN, 1990). This includes emergency medical care for the preservation of their life or the avoidance of irreparable harm to their health (Article 28). The CRMW contains migrant workers' rights to health-related information in a language and format that they comprehend, safe work conditions, and access to health care in immigration detention. The CRMW acknowledges that migrant workers often lack access to health care, especially undocumented migrants and migrant sex workers, and holds that states have the duty to protect non-citizens' right to health (Articles 43 and 45). The CRMW prohibits states from denying access to health care to migrants, including undocumented migrants or asylum seekers. States should take measures to address the underlying conditions of health such as migrant workers' human rights to housing, food, and civil and political rights, especially freedom from forced labor.

Special Rapporteur on the Right to Health

Paul Hunt from New Zealand served as the first Special Rapporteur on the Right of Everyone to the Enjoyment of the Highest Attainable Standard of Physical and Mental Health from 2002 to 2008. Hunt was appointed for his health activism to promote the right to health as a fundamental human right. The Special Rapporteur's role is to set the agenda for health rights, call attention to pressing issues, and receive complaints. Examples of individual complaints to the Special Rapporteur have included lack of access to health care, forced feeding of detainees or prisoners, persecution of health care professionals, discrimination against people based on their health status, forced medical treatment and sterilizations, abuse of psychiatric patients, poor conditions in psychiatric institutions, and denials of health care to migrant workers. Summaries of cases on these and additional topics along with replies from states can be accessed through the UN Office of the High Commissioner for Human Rights website. Other special rapporteurs also have connection to health rights, such as the special rapporteurs on education, food, adequate housing, and violence against women.

Exceptions during emergencies

There is a precedent for limiting civil and political rights during public health emergencies. Raising the debate on indivisibility, the Siracusa Principles represent international consensus for prioritizing the right to health in times of epidemic or disaster over rights to assembly or movement (UN, 1984). Limiting certain rights (some rights can never be abridged, such as freedom from torture, freedom of thought or religion) in emergencies should only be considered a last resort. These exceptions must be lawful, strictly necessary in the public interest, use the least restrictive measures, and not unreasonably arbitrary or discriminatory. An acceptable example is quarantine in the case of highly contagious and communicable disease (WHO, 2002).

Case studies of rights-based approaches to health

HealthRight International – Vietnam

HealthRight International is an NGO dedicated to realizing the human right to health (healthright.org). HealthRight was founded in 1990 by Jonathan Mann, a global champion of health and human rights, founding director of the Francois-Xavier Bagnoud Center for Health and Human Rights at Harvard University. Mann was also an early leader against the HIV/AIDS epidemic and the first director of the WHO's Global Programme on AIDS before his untimely death in an airplane crash en route to a WHO conference in 1998. HealthRight's mission is to build sustainable access to health through a rights-based approach. They partner with excluded communities to build local capacity for inclusive health systems. HealthRight works with a range of international partners including UN agencies (such as UNICEF and UN Women), USAID, academic units (NYU), private corporations (such as Johnson & Johnson and Boeing), and local NGOs (such as Ukrainian Foundation for Public Health and Sobon Support Group-Kenya). The populations that HealthRight works with include children and adolescents, people in conflict with the law, people living with HIV, people who use drugs, women, torture survivors, and semi-nomadic rural pastoralists. HealthRight has worked in North America, Eastern Europe, Africa, and Asia. HealthRight's rights-based approach includes capacity building, service delivery, advocacy, and research. Capacity building means training and education for social workers and other health personnel, facility improvement for health infrastructure, and community mobilization. HealthRight engages local health and social services delivery to target excluded populations with high quality, accessible, and acceptable health services. HealthRight trains health professionals to advocate with their clients, and lobbies states and health providers on nondiscrimination and participation in the right to health.

HealthRight has worked in Vietnam since 2010 on HIV/AIDS, violence prevention, and child welfare. HealthRight aims to halt the spread of HIV/AIDS in Vietnam, to prevent discrimination against those living with HIV, and to ensure their access to care. Combining care, support, and advocacy, HealthRight and its partners provides a comprehensive response to orphans and other children affected by HIV/AIDS, preventing institutionalization and abandonment. HealthRight's main partner in Vietnam is the Research and Training Centre for Community Development (RTCCD) (www.rtccd.org.vn/index.php/en). This local NGO was founded in 1996 and builds capacity through training and research for community health interventions which are the basis for advocacy for health policy reform. HealthRight and RTCCD jointly operate the Social Work Professional Development Centre, to provide training for social workers and para-social workers in Vietnam on practice skills for working with health, mental health, and child welfare. Training Vietnamese social workers revealed gaps in social work education, which led HealthRight to advocate for further professionalization of social work in Vietnam.

Treatment Action Campaign – South Africa

Treatment Action Campaign (TAC) is a coalition of individuals and organizations working on equitable and affordable access to HIV/AIDS treatment (www.tac. org.za/). Founded in 1998, TAC is well known among the Global South's civil society NGOs for its campaign resulting in South Africa's universal AIDS treatment program (Heywood, 2003; Heywood, 2009; UN, 2008). TAC utilized social mobilization, advocacy, and judicial litigation in realizing the right to health to ensure equal access to HIV/AIDS treatment. When in 2001 the South African government restricted the universal distribution of nevirapine, a medicine preventing mother-to-child HIV/AIDS transmission, to two research sites despite evidence that the drug was already effective, HIV-positive women without private insurance and/or access to the research sites could not afford nevirapine. TAC filed a legal complaint, contending that the government should provide access to nevirapine to all pregnant women in public hospitals. They argued the state violated the right to health which requires equitable access to medical resources. The case went to the South African Constitutional Court, which ruled in favor of TAC (Minister of Health v. Treatment Action Campaign, 2002). The court found the policy to be discriminatory against the poor, and mandated the state to progressively realize the right to health of pregnant women and their newborn children through a comprehensive and coordinated plan within existing resources. This led to the development of universal programs to reduce mother-to-child transmissions of HIV/AIDS.

Inter-American Commission on Human Rights – El Salvador

The Inter-American Commission on Human Rights (IACHR) is a regional human rights mechanism, guided by the Protocol of San Salvador, which receives complaints on the right to health (UN, 2008). In 2000, a submission was made by 27 people diagnosed with HIV/AIDS. They alleged that El Salvador violated their right to health by not providing triple-therapy treatment for HIV/AIDS. The IACHR found this to be a violation of their rights to life and health, and recommended that El Salvador provide triple-therapy, hospital, pharmaceutical, and nutritional care. The Supreme Court and legislature of El Salvador followed this recommendation with a legal order to provide care and a new national HIV/AIDS treatment policy (Jorge Odir Miranda Cortez et al. v. El Salvador, 2001).

People's Health Movement – India

The People's Health Movement is an international grassroots network of health promoters, professionals and activists organizing to address violations of health rights (www.phmovement.org). The movement engages in international and national campaigns for the right to health (Nadkarni & Vikram, 2009). Their approach incorporates people as active agents in their health, not passive recipients of health care. The rights-based principle of participation influences the movement's priority of bottom-up health planning. The movement's goal is to achieve broad and sustainable health initiatives rather than narrow policies that fail to impact overall population health outcomes. They seek to encourage health care systems that address the social determinants of health and mitigate the negative impact of globalization upon people's health. The People's Health Movement has national subgroups, such as India's Jan Swasthya Abhiyan (www.phmovement.org/india) which partner with social workers to document abuses of health rights and utilize public forums to pressure stakeholders for health rights. The Indian Right to Food movement employed similar tactics to achieve the provision of cooked meals for all primary school children in public schools.

Rights-based approaches to social work practice in health

Rights-based approaches incorporate the practice principles of dignity, nondiscrimination, participation, transparency, and accountability to ensure people's enjoyment of the right to health (WHO, 2002; Zuniga, Marks & Gostin, 2013). Social work practice that advances the right to health should work towards sustainable, health-promoting environments, equal access to health resources, and an adequate minimum standard of living (IFSW, 2012). Rights-based approaches to health require that health care be available, nondiscriminatory, culturally competent, and of high scientific and technological quality. The right to health includes preventative measures such as access to contraception and family planning, reducing accidents, immunizations against infections, preventing the spread of disease, supplying adequate water, basic sanitation infrastructure, protecting populations from exposure to hazards such as radiation or chemicals, and regulating and monitoring working conditions in industrial work sites. This also includes the duty to prevent harmful cultural practices that violate the right to health.

Social workers in health settings and other health professionals have an indispensable role in promoting the right to health (Hunt, 2003). Rights-based social work practice in health integrates micro and macro levels of intervention, including individual medical and structural public health strategies. Rights-based approaches to social work practice in health should draw upon the person-in-environment perspective to balance the right to health prevention and treatment among people with the right to the underlying determinants that influence health. Rights-based social work practice should combine individual case advocacy in both clinical and non-clinical settings, policy practice, advocacy, lobbying, social pedagogy and community education strategies, social development, and research and education in local and global contexts (Nadkarni & Vikram, 2009).

Rights-based approaches to health add value to social work practice by re-conceptualizing health from a welfare outcome, a charitable construct, or a market commodity into a human right. This strengthens the justification for social work practice in health settings by grounding it in international standards. This is an important counterargument to economic cost-saving rationales in favor of restricting poor people's access to health care (Farmer, 2005). Rights-based approaches prioritize the health needs of communities with the worst health outcomes, such as those living in poverty (Farmer, 2001). Social workers can affirm the dignity of people with health issues by treating others with interpersonal empathy and compassion and kindness (Wronka, 2008). Respect for the dignity and privacy of individuals can facilitate more sensitive and humane care, resulting in better prevention and treatment (Grodin, Tarantola, Annas & Gruskin, 2013).

Social workers in health settings have the right to health as well (Beletsky, Ezer, Overall, Byrne & Cohen, 2013). This includes the right to quality working conditions, the right to free association, and the right to conscientious objection to perform procedures that violate their morals, ethics, or values. Health care practitioners' rights are violated when they are pressured to deny treatment to certain individuals or groups, to break confidentiality, and to conceal human rights violations (Allhoff, 2008).

Rights-based approaches should be based on nondiscrimination; discrimination and stigma of people with health conditions can limit health interventions and contribute to ill health. Practitioners should ensure that health policies and programs are rigorously evaluated for biases toward excluding typically vulnerable populations such as women and children, people with disabilities, indigenous people, racial, ethnic, religious, linguistic, or sexual minorities, displaced people and migrants – especially undocumented migrants – and people living with HIV/AIDS.

Participation and inclusion for rights-based approaches to health means that people have meaningful input into health interventions that affect them, including access to information, the decision-making process, and the design, delivery, and evaluation of programs. This helps to ensure that health policies and programs are responsive to the people they serve. Clinical practice should involve people's participation, input, and decision making in any treatment planning. Practitioners can use assessment and information gathering tools to monitor and explore health patterns such as diet and exercise, and other health behaviors.

Transparency means practitioners should analyze health policies and programs from a human rights perspective, investigating how they impact and influence the right to health, as well as the health consequences of human rights violations (Nadkarni & Vikram, 2009). Social workers practicing in health settings have the opportunity and obligation to witness and document human rights violations (Orbinski, Beyrer & Singh, 2007).

Health indicators are another important facet of rights-based approaches to health, and can yield significant transparency for social work practice. Health indicators help to operationalize health practices and can illuminate how health interacts with other factors, including health care policies and programs and social determinants of health (UN, 2000; WHO, 2008). Health indicators can bring rights-based approaches to health in line with the evidence-based model of health. Indicators can be structural, process, or outcome-related assessments of institutions, facilities, policies, and participation. Structural indicators refer to a state's acceptance of international health and human rights standards, such as signing or ratifying agreements. Process indicators refer to policies related to state obligations to the right to health, for example training and providing a professional workforce, also reflected in health indicators such as the number of childbirths attended by skilled health personnel. Outcome indicators refer to the result of health care policies and programs and conditions of health priority areas within the population, such as the maternal health ratio.

Rights-based health practice means that social workers must be transparent about assessing and protecting people from abusive medical practices. Social workers must protect people's right to be free from non-consensual medical treatment and experimentation and the right to sexual and reproductive health (Hunt, 2006; UN, 2000). Rights-based social work practice incorporates human rights into the design, delivery, monitoring, and evaluation of health services (Gruskin, Mills & Tarantola, 2007). Social workers should also support transparent guidelines for accrediting medical facilities, personnel, and equipment. A rights-based agenda for health should prioritize new research and education programs (Farmer, 2005).

Transparency and accountability in rights-based approaches to health means that health policies and programs be subject to international and domestic law, judicial and administrative review, political oversight, and reporting and watchdog groups. Holding duty-bearers accountable for the right to health requires advocacy. Rights-based approaches to health must surpass traditional human rights campaign strategies of naming and shaming, letter writing, and media coverage and include indicators, benchmarks, impact assessments, and budgetary analysis (Hunt, 2007). Social workers should support the development of national health policies, participatory budgeting, monitoring tools such as rights-based indicators, regulatory frameworks with assessments, and accountability. Judicial mechanisms that provide individual redress after violations of the right to health are equally important. Education programs in schools and communities can foster healthy behaviors and encourage people's awareness and attainment of the right to health.

Human rights-based approaches to health can address power relations that contribute to human rights violations. Empowering civil society and communities to claim their right to health is a pillar of global health (Friedman & Gostin, 2012; Gostin et al., 2013; Hunt, 2006). Social workers should lobby for accessible and affordable health care and for the underlying determinants of health. Globally, social workers should support the equitable distribution of health technology and benefits of medical research, promoting access to healthy foods that are appropriately priced and culturally appropriate. Research should be conducted to determine the outcomes and efficacy of these interventions (Wronka, 2008). Social workers can utilize rights-based indicators, benchmarks, impact assessments, and budgetary analysis to promote accountability for the right to health (UN, 2008).

Taken together, rights-based approaches to health should result in increased capacity among duty-bearers and rights-holders. Health policymakers, health administrators and practitioners, and industry regulators are responsible for non-interfering and protecting people's right to health through legislative, judicial, administrative, budgetary, and regulatory measures. Individual rights-holders should be empowered to understand and access their right to health.

For further reading on rights-based approaches to health

Amnesty International Health Network

Advocating for health care-related human rights.
http://healthandhumanrightsproject.com/

François-Xavier Bagnoud Center for Health and Human Rights and Harvard School of Public Health

An academic center focused on health and human rights through research, teaching, and international collaborations for service and policy development.
http://fxb.harvard.edu/

Health and Human Rights Journal

An online, open-access academic publication fostering dialogue among health and human rights practitioners.
www.hhrjournal.org/

Médicins Sans Frontières / Doctors Without Borders

A private international association of health care workers providing assistance to populations in distress, recipient of the 1999 Nobel Peace Prize.
www.doctorswithoutborders.org/

Physicians for Human Rights

An NGO using science and medicine to stop human rights violations, partner recipient of the 1997 Nobel Peace Prize with the International Campaign to Ban Landmines.
http://physiciansforhumanrights.org/

Special Rapporteur on the Right of Everyone to the Enjoyment of the Highest Attainable Standard of Physical and Mental Health

Independent expert appointed by the Human Rights Council monitoring the right to health worldwide.
www.ohchr.org/EN/Issues/Health/Pages/SRRightHealthIndex.aspx

UN Office of the High Commissioner for Human Rights – Toolkit on the Right to Health

The Toolkit on the Right to Health has resources on the key aspects, normative framework, relevant mechanisms, publications, and special issues related to the right to health.
www.ohchr.org/EN/Issues/ESCR/Pages/Health.aspx

World Health Organization – health and human rights

Resources on many health and human rights topics and organizations.
www.who.int/hhr/links/en/

References

Allhoff, F. (Ed.). (2008). *Physicians at war: The dual-loyalties challenge.* Dordrecht: Springer.

Amon, J. (2010). *Abusing patients: Health providers' complicity in torture and cruel, inhuman or degrading treatment.* In Human Rights Watch (HRW) *World Report 2010* (pp. 49–59). New York: HRW. Retrieved from: www.hrw.org/sites/default/files/related_material/patients_0.pdf

Beletsky, L., Ezer, T., Overall, J., Byrne, I., & Cohen, J. (2013). *Advancing human rights in patient care: The law in seven transitional countries.* Open Society Foundations. Retrieved from: www.opensocietyfoundations.org/sites/default/files/Advancing-Human-Rights-in-Patient-Care-20130516.pdf

Claude, R., & Weston, B. (Eds.). (2006). *Human rights in the world community: Issues and action* (3rd ed.). Philadelphia: University of Pennsylvania Press.

Farmer, P. (2001). The major infectious diseases in the world – to treat or not to treat? *New England Journal of Medicine, 345*(3), 208–210.

Farmer, P. (2005). *Pathologies of power: Health, human rights, and the new war on the poor.* Berkeley: University of California Press.

Fewtrell, L., Pruss-Ustun, A., Bos, R., Gore, F., & Bartram, J. (2007). *Water, sanitation, and hygiene: Quantifying the health impact at national and local levels in countries with incomplete water supply and sanitation coverage.* Environmental Burden of Disease Series No. 15. Geneva: WHO. Retrieved from: http://whqlibdoc.who.int/publications/2007/9789241595759_eng.pdf

Friedman, E., & Gostin, O. (2012). Pillars for progress on the right to health: Harnessing the potential of human rights through a framework convention on global health. *Health & Human Rights, 14*(1), 4–19.

Gambrill, E. (2006). Evidence-based practice and policy: Choices ahead. *Research on Social Work Practice, 16*(3), 338–357.

Gostin, L., Friedman, E., Buse, K., Waris, A., Mulumba, M., Joel, M., . . . Sridhar, D. (2013). Towards a Framework Convention on Global Health. *Bulletin of the World Health Organization, 91*, 790–793. Retrieved from: www.who.int/bulletin/volumes/91/10/12–114447/en/

Grodin, M., Tarantola, D., Annas, G., & Gruskin, S. (Eds.). (2013). *Health and human rights in a changing world.* New York: Routledge.

Gruskin, S., Mills, E., & Tarantola, D. (2007). History, principles and practice of health and human rights. *Lancet, 370*, 449–455.

Heywood, M. (2003). Current developments: Preventing mother-to-child HIV transmission in South Africa: Background, strategies and outcomes of the Treatment Action Campaign's case against the Minister of Health. *South African Journal of Human Rights, 19*(2), 278–315.

Heywood, M. (2009). South Africa's Treatment Action Campaign: Combining law and social mobilization to realize the right to health. *Journal of Human Rights Practice, 1*(1), 14–36.

Hunt, P. (2003). The UN Special Rapporteur on the right to health: Key objectives, themes, and interventions. *Health and Human Rights, 7*, 1–27.

Hunt, P. (2006). *Report of the Special Rapporteur on the right of everyone to the enjoyment of the highest attainable standard of physical and mental health.* New York: UN Office of the High Commissioner for Human Rights. Retrieved from: http://daccess-dds-ny.un.org/doc/UNDOC/GEN/G06/114/69/PDF/G0611469.pdf?OpenElement

Hunt, P. (2007). Right to the highest attainable standard of health. *Lancet, 370*, 369–371.

International Federation of Social Workers (IFSW). (2012). *Policy Statement – Health.* Berne: Author. Retrieved from: http://ifsw.org/policies/health/

Jorge Odir Miranda Cortez et al. v. El Salvador. (2001). Report No. 29/11. Case 12.249. Inter-American Commission on Human Rights. Retrieved from: www1.umn.edu/humanrts/cases/29–01.html

Mann, J. (1997). Medicine and public health, ethics, and human rights. *Hastings Center Report, 27*(3), 6–13.

Minister of Health v. Treatment Action Campaign. (2002). 5 SA 721 (CC) (South Africa).

Nadkarni, V., & Vikram, K. (2009). The right to health: Illusion or possibility? In P. Bywaters, E. McLeod, & L. Napier (Eds.), *Social work and global health inequalities: Practice and policy developments* (pp. 23–36). Bristol: Policy Press.

Orbinski, J., Beyrer, C., & Singh, S. (2007). Violations of human rights: Health practitioners as witnesses. *Lancet, 370*(9588), 25–31.

Physicians for Human Rights (PHR). (2008). *Broken laws, broken lives: Medical evidence of torture by US personnel and its impact.* Cambridge, MA: Author. Retrieved from: https://s3.amazonaws.com/PHR_Reports/BrokenLaws_14.pdf

Richmond, M. (1917). *Social diagnosis.* New York: Russell Sage Foundation.

United Nations (UN). (1948). Universal Declaration of Human Rights. UN General Assembly. 10 December, 1948. Retrieved from: www.un.org/Overview/rights.htm

United Nations (UN). (1965). *International Convention on the Elimination of All Forms of Racial Discrimination.* New York: Author. Retrieved from: www.ohchr.org/EN/ProfessionalInterest/Pages/CERD.aspx

United Nations (UN). (1966a). *International Covenant on Civil and Political Rights.* New York: Author. Retrieved from: www.ohchr.org/en/professionalinterest/pages/ccpr.aspx

United Nations (UN). (1966b). *International Covenant on Economic, Social and Cultural Rights.* New York: Author. Retrieved from: www.ohchr.org/EN/ProfessionalInterest/Pages/CESCR.aspx

United Nations (UN). (1979). *Convention on the Elimination of All Forms of Discrimination Against Women.* New York: Author. Retrieved from: www.un.org/womenwatch/daw/cedaw/text/econvention.htm

United Nations (UN). (1984). *The Siracusa Principles on the limitation and derogation provisions in the International Covenant on Civil and Political Rights.* New York: UN Commission on Human Rights. Retrieved from: www1.umn.edu/humanrts/instree/siracusaprinciples.html

United Nations (UN). (1989). *Convention on the Rights of the Child.* New York: Author. Retrieved from: www.ohchr.org/en/professionalinterest/pages/crc.aspx

United Nations (UN). (1990). *Convention on the Rights of Migrant Workers and Their Families.* New York: Author. Retrieved from: www2.ohchr.org/english/bodies/cmw/cmw.htm

United Nations (UN). (2000). *General Comment No. 14: The right to the highest attainable standard of health (Art. 12).* New York: UN Committee on Economic, Social and Cultural Rights. Retrieved from: http://tbinternet.ohchr.org/_layouts/treatybodyexternal/Download.aspx?symbolno=E%2fC.12%2f2000%2f4&Lang=en

United Nations (UN). (2006). *Convention on the Rights of People with Disabilities.* New York: Author. Retrieved from: www.un.org/disabilities/convention/conventionfull.shtml

United Nations (UN). (2008). *Fact Sheet No. 31: The Right to Health.* Geneva: UN Office of the High Commissioner for Human Rights. Retrieved from: www.ohchr.org/Documents/Publications/Factsheet31.pdf

World Health Organization (WHO). (1946). *Constitution of the World Health Organization.* Geneva: Author. Retrieved from: http://apps.who.int/gb/bd/PDF/bd47/EN/constitution-en.pdf

World Health Organization (WHO). (2002, July 1). *25 questions and answers on health and human rights.* Health & Human Rights Publication Series. Geneva: Author. Retrieved from: www.who.int/hhr/NEW37871OMSOK.pdf

World Health Organization (WHO). (2008). *Closing the gap in a generation: Health equity through action on the social determinants of health.* Commission on the Social Determinants of Health Final Report. Geneva: Author. Retrieved from: http://whqlibdoc.who.int/publications/2008/9789241563703_eng.pdf

World Health Organization (WHO). (2013). *Fact Sheet No. 323: The Right to Health.* Geneva: Author. Retrieved from: www.who.int/mediacentre/factsheets/fs323/en/

Wronka, J. (2008). *Human rights and social justice: Social action and service for the helping and health professions.* Thousand Oaks, CA: Sage.

Zuniga, J., Marks, S., & Gostin, L. (Eds.). (2013). *Advancing the human right to health.* Oxford: Oxford University Press.

7

HUMAN RIGHTS-BASED APPROACHES TO MENTAL HEALTH

Mental health is a key component of overall good health (WHO, 2013). Mental health matters; there can be no health without mental health. Mental health is a neglected aspect of the right to health, rarely included in the global health discourse and the human rights agenda (Burns, 2013).

One quarter of the world's population will experience a mental disorder in their lifetime (WHO, 2001). This is amplified during environmental disasters, humanitarian crises, political instability, armed conflict, violence, and terrorism, which increase the burden of stress upon the general population resulting in increased distress. An estimated 450 million people globally suffer from some form of mental disorder (Burns, 2013; Hunt, 2005). Mental disability is correlated with disproportionate rates of disability and mortality (WHO, 2013). The chance of premature death is 40 to 60% greater for persons with major depression and schizophrenia. Depression is the largest cause of disability worldwide representing 4.3% of the total disease burden and 11% of all years lived with disability. A majority of those who commit suicide have a mental disability; suicide is the second most common cause of death for young people globally. Although the true prevalence of mental disability is obscured by stigma and lack of data, available evidence indicates that lower and middle-income countries in the Global South bear a disproportionate share of the population with mental disability (Burns, 2013). An estimated two thirds of people with mental disabilities live in the Global South. The suicide rate is highest in the Global South.

Mental health can be understood to be the ability to function productively, cope with the normal stresses of life, achieve one's human development, and contribute to one's community (Burns, 2013; WHO, 2013). Mental health means having the means and opportunity to meaningfully participate in society. Mental health is determined by a combination of individual factors, including the capacity for self-management of emotion, cognition, behavior, and social relationships, and also with larger, external, macro factors such as social, cultural, economic, political, and environmental considerations in additional to social policies, social protections, standards of living, working conditions, and community supports. People with mental disability are negatively affected by structural factors such as poverty, inequality, homelessness, and discrimination.

Despite the widespread scope of mental disability, very few people are receiving care (Hunt, 2005). While 50 to 65% of people with mental disabilities are estimated to be untreated, in the Global South it is estimated to be between 76 and 85% (Burns, 2013; WHO, 2013). In 2001, most states in the Global South spent less than 1% of their health budgets on mental health (WHO, 2011), evidencing a distinct lack of parity. Globally, annual mental health spending is less than $2 per person; in low-income countries it is less than $0.25 (WHO, 2013). The estimated burden of mental disability globally is 13% yet only 3% of global spending is for mental health. Sixty-seven percent of this spending is accounted for in mental hospitals, which are frequently associated with poor clinical outcomes and risk of human rights violations and thus considered to be an outdated mode of treatment (WHO, 2013). Over 40% of the world's nations lack a national mental health policy; over 90% of countries in the world have no child and adolescent mental health policy. Where mental health services are available in the Global South, often out-of-pocket fees are required. This underscores the lack of access to affordable mental health care; health insurance often does not cover mental health services (Hunt, 2005). The global mental health workforce, including social workers, is grossly insufficient (Burns, 2013; WHO, 2013). Roughly half the world lives in countries with significantly limited access to mental health practitioners (WHO, 2013).

In states where mental health care is available, it is often substandard and inadequate, predominantly centralized into large institutions such as psychiatric hospitals, without significant community-based alternatives (Hunt, 2005). Although the last decade indicates a slow decrease in institutional care, globally 63% of psychiatric beds are in mental hospitals, which receive 67% of the mental health expenditures (WHO, 2013). Outpatient mental health services are 58 times more prevalent in high-income versus low-income countries (WHO, 2013). Only 49% of low-income countries have mental health service-user or consumer organizations, whereas 83% of high-income countries do (WHO, 2013). Institutional facilities typically segregate people from the community and public, at greater risk of human rights violations (Hunt, 2005).

The international human rights community uses the term mental disability to refer to psychiatric disorders (mental illness, mood, and thought disorders) and developmental disabilities (intellectual disabilities, brain damage, genetic abnormalities) (Hunt, 2005). The term "disability" connects mental health to disability rights and refers to either permanent or temporary limitations, restrictions, or impairments in one's activities or participation and is influenced by the interaction between individual characteristics and the social environment (WHO, 2013). People with mental disabilities have a range of mental, emotional, behavioral, and physical abilities, as do all humans. In some cases, their abilities may be limited.

However, a rights-based approach takes the view that it is the discrimination that people with disabilities face, discrimination resulting from stigma of their condition, that constitutes their disability status (Burns, 2013; Hunt, 2005; Oliver, 2009). It is the complex interplay between individual factors (genetic, neurological, and others) and social factors (such as culture, religion, discrimination, and stigma) that results in the condition of disability and compromises human rights. This is similar to the dynamic in the right to health, and illuminates why this human right is identified as the right to the highest attainable standard of health, instead of a right to be healthy. It is the disability-based stigma that leads people with mental disabilities to face violations of their rights and social exclusion in the areas of health, housing, education, work and poverty, social security, and denials of their fundamental freedoms of liberty, privacy, and self-determination (Hunt, 2005). Social, economic, and political factors shape the experience of mental disability and the nature of the service system that people may or may not access. People with mental disabilities are exceptionally vulnerable to human rights violations. They suffer from discrimination and exclusion in society, and often in care they are also at jeopardy.

Traditional approaches to mental health

Mental disability has been acknowledged as a special affliction since ancient times, drawing the compassion of Indian Emperor Ashoka and Roman Emperor Marcus Aurelius. However, mental illness has historically been associated with non-conformity with moral, social, cultural, or political values. Extreme examples include the diagnosis of drapetomania, a disorder causing slaves to run away, in the southern U.S. during the 1800s, and the inclusion of the diagnosis of homosexuality in the DSM until the last few decades.

Traditional practice in the field of mental health has paralleled the foibles of the medical field. Early policies were characterized by exclusion and punishment. Reforms attempted to integrate scientific and humanitarian advances, resulting in the moral treatment and mental hygiene movements. Concern for human rights, treatment efficacy, and cost containment led to widespread deinstitutionalization in favor of community-based care. However, at least in the U.S., the promise of community-based alternatives for people with mental disability was not realized, and the population increasingly became homeless and incarcerated (Torrey, 2013).

Contemporary practice in the field of mental health remains heavily influenced by the medical model, which emphasizes the assessment, diagnosis, and treatment of individuals (Dudley, Silove & Gale, 2012). Continued concern for cost efficiency has led to managed care, brief time-limited interventions, and symptom management shaping mental health treatment. People with mental disabilities have been traditionally viewed as disempowered and passive, in need of intervention. Traditional models reinforce patterns of paternalism, charity, and powerlessness of the "patient" (Burns, 2013; Oliver, 2009). In this model, the person with a mental disability is in need of a medical solution – from the medical perspective, all problems are medical and not necessarily political, social, or cultural. However, the medical approach, even the genetic and biomedical advances that strengthen this approach, and the public health approach are insufficient unless they can recognize and incorporate the social forces that interact with the individual ones (Burns, 2013).

Social workers are critically involved in the field of mental health. It is estimated that social workers provide almost half of all mental health services in the U.S., and this is projected to grow (CSWE, 2011). In some rural areas and under served communities, social workers may be the only mental health professionals present. Social work has the potential to bridge the individually focused fields of medicine and psychology with social, economic, and political reforms. However, social work has also emphasized illness, labeling, and deficits, reinforcing the worst of the medical model in mental health. Some evidence suggests that the medical model is the dominant frame in social work education when it comes to mental health, and that students are unprepared to work with people with severe mental disability (Starnino, 2009).

The human right to mental health

Mental health and human rights are rarely connected (Dudley, Silove & Gale, 2012; Gostin & Gable, 2004). The right to mental health is a core aspect of the right to health. The right to health identifies mental health as on par with physical health. Mental health rights have recently been included with disability rights, which may contribute to the equal treatment of people with mental disability (Morrissey, 2012). The rights of people with mental disability are indivisible, including civil, political, economic, social, and cultural rights. The concept of indivisibility relates to the importance of underlying determinants for mental health. The enjoyment of other human rights can reduce stress, anxiety, discrimination, and depression and form the basis for the underlying determinants of mental health (Gable & Gostin, 2009). In reality, mental health is significantly related to human rights. Human rights violations can harm mental health. Mental health policies can violate human rights. Positive mental health can reinforce human rights.

Non-binding instruments

These three instruments represent important developments in the evolution of international consensus. These affirm the principles of dignity, nondiscrimination, participation, transparency, and accountability and can be used to interpret and advocate for international human rights standards regarding mental health.

Principles for the protection of persons with mental illness and for the improvement of mental health care (MI Principles)

In 1991 the UN adopted the Mental Illness Principles representing current international consensus of standards for mental health care, treatment, and the rights of people in mental health facilities (Hunt, 2005; Rosenthal & Rubenstein, 1993;

UN, 1991). The MI Principles prohibit discrimination on the grounds of mental illness, as stigma negatively impacts access to care and affects the rights to employment, adequate housing, education, and more. These principles affirmed the rights to medication, informed consent to treatment, to treatment in the least restrictive environment, and to community integration and care, as far as possible, in the community in which one lives. The 1991 MI Principles were an important step in the international recognition of the rights of people with mental disabilities. However, it has been criticized by human rights organizations and advocacy groups such as the World Network of Users and Survivors of Psychiatry (2001) for supporting the medical model, endorsing involuntary detention and coercive treatment, inadequate protections of informed consent, diluting the right to community with the qualifier "as far as possible", and for development without consultation from people with mental disabilities (Hunt, 2005).

Standard Rules on the Equalization of Opportunities for Persons with Disabilities (Standard Rules)

In 1993 the UN adopted the Standard Rules, which contain 22 commitments to health care, rehabilitation, support, awareness-raising, education, employment, family life, and policy development and emphasis on the participation of people with mental disabilities and their representative organizations (Hunt, 2005; UN, 1993). Although not legally enforceable, the Standard Rules have encouraged many states to pass disability legislation.

Montreal Declaration on Intellectual Disability

In 2004 the international community adopted the Montreal Declaration on Intellectual Disability at a Pan-American Health Organization and WHO conference (Lecompt & Mercier, 2007). This landmark recognition of the rights of persons with intellectual disabilities included the right to mental health.

Madrid International Plan of Action on Ageing (MIPAA)

The 2002 MIPAA addressed the mental health of older adults under the priority area of advancing health and well-being (UN, 2002). MIPAA calls for the development of comprehensive mental health care services, including prevention, early intervention, treatment, and management of mental health problems in older adults.

Human rights treaties

The International Covenant on Civil and Political Rights prohibits degrading treatment or punishment and requires informed consent for medical or scientific experimentation. The International Covenant on Economic, Social and Cultural Rights recognizes the right of everyone to the highest attainable standard of mental health.

The Convention on the Rights of the Child mandates the right to a full and decent life, with dignity and active participation in the community for children with mental or physical disability (Gostin & Gable, 2004).

Several general comments and recommendations have expanded upon the right to mental health. General Comment No. 5 (GC 5) includes the right to mental health among the rights of persons with disabilities and prohibits discrimination on the basis of mental health or mental disability (UN, 1994). GC 5 also affirms that states, as duty-bearers of the right to mental health, are required to establish institutions, equitably distributed throughout the country, that provide mental health services. States are also required to ensure for the proper training of mental health practitioners and for a sufficient workforce to staff the necessary hospitals, clinics, and health-related facilities. General Comment No. 14 (GC 14) interprets the right to appropriate mental health treatment, care, facilities, and goods (UN, 2000). GC 14 discusses the controversial exception to prohibited coercive treatment in the case of mental illness. GC 14 stipulates that exceptions should be restricted and made in line with best practices and international standards. General Recommendation 27 urges that comprehensive health care policies should encompass behavioral interventions and lifestyle changes such as healthy nutritional practices and active living, and attend to the mental and emotional needs of older women, especially those with disabilities and from minority groups (UN, 2010).

Convention on the Rights of Persons with Disabilities (CRPD)

After the Declaration on the Rights of Disabled Persons in 1975, the UN General Assembly adopted the World Program of Action concerning Disabled Persons in 1982 and declared a UN Decade for Disabled Persons (Gostin & Gable, 2004). The CRPD, adopted in 2006, was an evolution beyond the traditional medical model of disability and consistent with a rights-based perspective, and does not define mental disability in biological terms, but broadly as a long-term mental, intellectual, or sensory impairment which, combined with social barriers, limits someone's participation in society (UN, 2006).

The CRPD contains the right to the highest attainable standard of health (Article 25) and contains the principles of human dignity (Article 1), nondiscrimination, participation, equality of opportunity, and accessibility (Article 3). Respecting the dignity of people with disabilities requires embracing their full humanity as subjects with self-determination. Key rights include the right to participate in decisions that affect their well-being, to give their own free consent, and to be active and productive participants in society. Nondiscrimination means that people with disabilities are entitled to the same range, quality, and standard of care as other people. States are responsible for combating stereotypes and prejudice against people with disabilities (Article 8) and supporting equal protection under the law, protecting people's self-determination and from paternalistic and restrictive policies, and involuntary institutionalization (Article 12). The CRPD requires that people with disabilities have the support necessary to exercise their legal capacity and fulfill their right to participate.

Access to health and social services necessary due to disability is a key principle of the CRPD, across physical, financial, and other barriers (Articles 25 and 26). This can include early identification and intervention, services designed to minimize and prevent further disabilities as well as orthopedic and rehabilitation services to facilitate independence, social and community integration, and prevent further disability. CRPD holds that people in rural or slum areas, or who may lack affordable care, have the same right to accessible and affordable care as anyone else. States are obligated to provide services within geographical proximity to people with disabilities. The CRPD contains the right of people with disabilities to reasonable accommodations, which are modifications and adjustments not imposing a disproportionate burden, that are necessary for the enjoyment of rights and freedoms on an equal basis with others. Additionally the CRPD contains the rights of people with disability to movement, mobility, independent living, and full inclusion within the community including full access to and participation in cultural life, recreation, leisure, and sport. The CRPD also requires medical, health, and social work professionals to be trained in the ethical standards of informed consent.

Special Rapporteur on the Right to Health

The Special Rapporteur on the Right of Everyone to the Enjoyment of the Highest Attainable Standard of Physical and Mental Health issued a special report elaborating on human rights and mental health issues (Hunt, 2005). People with mental disabilities, more likely to suffer poverty and deprivation, are entitled to medical, health, and mental health care and supportive services as well as to the underlying determinants of health. These rights pertain especially to those inside psychiatric hospitals and facilities (Hunt, 2005).

The report clarifies that the right to mental health includes freedoms, such as the right to be free from discrimination and interference in one's body and health, including abuses such as forced sterilization, rape, and other forms of sexual violence. The right to mental health includes the fundamental freedom to be in control of one's own body and health. The MI Principles acknowledge exceptional circumstances in which people can be involuntarily committed to a hospital or psychiatric facility. The Special Rapporteur has indicated that such violations of individual rights and freedoms require numerous procedural safeguards protecting against abuses of involuntary commitment, such as consultation from mental health professionals, safe and adequate facilities, judicial review, and access to complaint and redress mechanisms.

The Special Rapporteur has also clarified the obligations of duty-bearers under the right to mental health, including progressive realization and immediate effect. The progressive realization of the right to mental health under resource constraints requires that states make progress towards their goal, and that their expectations are matched to their means. The obligation of immediate effect means that states, regardless of resource constraints, are immediately obligated to ensure the right to be free from non-consensual treatment and non-discrimination.

Controversy in the right to mental health

The human right to mental health carries certain controversies surrounding involuntary commitment and coercive treatment. The controversy lies in the tension between the rights of the individual and of the community, between the right to be sick and the right to be well. The MI Principles were criticized by disability rights activists who were deeply opposed to coercive practices that, they maintain, violate the human rights of people with mental disabilities. Human rights standards recommend procedural protections of the person's self-determination that guarantees the rights to counsel, appeal, judicial review, and complaint and redress mechanisms for violations (Yamin & Rosenthal, 2005). Some prominent psychiatrists have defended the bio-psycho-medical model of mental health and have criticized the anti-psychiatry movement (Torrey, 1997). Their concern is that politically correct rhetoric and misguided protests prevents people from getting the help that they need, resulting in increased incidence of neglect, homelessness, and suicide. They view the freedom to be insane as a hoax that deceives people with mental disability.

Case studies of rights-based approaches to mental health

Mental Health Users Network of Zambia

The Mental Health Users Network of Zambia (MHUNZ) is a nonprofit membership organization representing people who have experienced mental distress (Katontoka, 2007; MDAC & MHUNZ, 2014; WHO, 2010). MHUNZ was identified as a best practice for building the capacity of people with mental and psychosocial issues to participate in public affairs (WHO, 2010). MHUNZ had 220 registered members in 2007. Users' networks are an emerging movement in Africa seeking to empower users to strengthen their identity and improve their situation. Users' networks in Kenya, South Africa, Tanzania, Uganda, and Zambia have conducted awareness-raising campaigns, self-help projects, and advocated for mental health services. The founder and president of MHUNZ, Sylvester Katontoka, is a mental health user who was hospitalized to prevent suicide. His experience included stigmatization, discrimination, isolated confinement, and degrading treatment in a facility with conditions violating international standards.

MHUNZ allows people with mental disabilities to come together for mutual support and information. MHUNZ combats stigma and discrimination in the wider society through its collaboration with the government, media, and international NGOs. MHUNZ engages in policy advocacy by identifying needs and lobbying for rights and services. Their advocacy has contributed to mental health policy reforms and their community organizing has led to the mobilization and sensitization of communities about mental health issues. MHUNZ also conducts awareness-raising and outreach on a regular radio program. In their direct work with people with mental disabilities, they conduct home visits and educate family members. In addition to lobbying on specific legislation, MHUNZ conducts education on the electoral process for people with mental disabilities to promote their participation in the political process and to amplify their influence on mental health policy. MHUNZ, in partnership with the Mental Disability Advocacy Center, conducted the first study on the experiences of people with mental disabilities in Zambia from a human rights perspective (MDAC & MHUNZ, 2014). Their report documented human rights violations against people with mental disabilities in their communities, by traditional healers, in the criminal justice system, and in mental health care.

MindFreedom International

MindFreedom International is a nonprofit coalition of over 100 grassroots organizations and thousands of members that promotes the human rights of people with mental disability (www.mindfreedom.org) (Minkowitz, Galves, Brown, Kovary & Remba, 2006; Oaks, 2007; Taylor, 2007; Wronka, 2008). Rooted in the 1970 psychiatric survivors' movement, ex-psychiatric patient groups such as the Insane Liberation Front, the Mental Patients Liberation Front, and dissident mental health professionals, MindFreedom International began as a newsletter in 1986 and coalesced while protesting the 1990 American Psychiatric Association's conference as the Support Coalition International which became MindFreedom International in 2005. Comprised of individuals affected by the mental health system, professionals, advocates, and family members, MindFreedom's vision is for a nonviolent revolution of freedom, equality, truth, and human rights for people affected by the mental health system, through their goals of challenging psychiatric abuse in medication or institutions, supporting self-determination of survivors and consumers, and promoting safe, humane, and effective mental health options.

MindFreedom is a civil society consultant to the UN Committee on Economic, Social and Cultural Rights. In 2006 MindFreedom, in collaboration with other advocacy groups, submitted a shadow report on psychiatric violations of human rights as part of the Disability Working Group to the Human Rights Committee, the monitoring body for the ICCPR. MindFreedom used their shadow report to highlight violations of the rights to be free from discrimination, torture or cruel, inhuman, or degrading punishment, and from coercion; as well as freedom of thought and equal protection under the law. This shadow report highlighted documented violations including the forced drugging with psychotropic medication of people with psychosocial disabilities, including prisoners held at Guantanamo Bay. It also called attention to gender and racial disparities in the administration of electroconvulsive therapy (ECT), and abuses and overuse of ECT to the detriment and harm of people with mental disabilities. MindFreedom also raised the issue of increased use of mental health screenings in schools of children. These screening instruments do not have evidence of their validity or reliability, and do not include informed consent. The use of inappropriate measures such as these contributes to overestimates of mental disability, and research conducted without children's meaningful consent is tied to the overuse of psychiatric medication among children (Gambrill, 2012). Often such unreliable screening tools are the product of pharmacological corporate research that, either intentionally or inadvertently, supports the wider use of psycho-pharmacological medication.

Shadow reports are a human rights tactic that combines research, media, and lobbying skills, often with organizing and coalition building, in preparing an alternative report to submit to human rights monitoring bodies. These reports, often submitted by civil society and advocacy NGOs, are alternatives to state reports and provide a shadow of the official record. In this capacity, shadow reports can be used to supplement or critique omissions in state reports. In addition to shadow reports, MindFreedom has also made a submission to the Committee against Torture for its consideration of the U.S. report on coercive psychiatric interventions and submitted comments to the U.S.'s periodic reports to the Committee on Civil and Political Rights.

BasicNeeds – Sri Lanka

BasicNeeds is an international nonprofit organization working to protect the human rights of people with mental disability and epilepsy in the Global South (www.basicneeds.org). In Sri Lanka, BasicNeeds developed a mental health and development model based on the principle of participation of people with mental disability (WHO, 2010). Community volunteers conduct community-based services, including monthly mental health camps that have increased outpatient services in collaboration with specialty hospitals, outreach clinics, and outpatient clinics for medication. A third of these volunteers are individuals who used to be service-users. People with mental disabilities see themselves as living case studies and encourage others through their own example and through mutual support.

BasicNeeds Sri Lanka has received national and international recognition for effective service delivery and as a model of community mental health. Their newsletter is staffed in part by people with mental disabilities. They apply social entrepreneurship in a sustainable livelihoods program for people with mental disability and their families. Programs educate members about family budgeting, reducing family conflict, and home gardening and horticulture therapy. They have also provided services to the victims of the tsunami disaster.

BasicNeeds operates horticulture farms in Sri Lanka, some on the grounds of psychiatric hospitals, that provide people with mental disability the opportunity to work. The workers are drawn from people who struggle to succeed in community-based vocational programs, typically having been institutionalized for years and facing extreme poverty. Typical work on the horticultural farms includes clearing land, raising beds, planting, preparing seed beds, watering, harvesting, or landscaping. The farms produce mushrooms, cabbage, peppers, onions, carrots, sweet peppers, and cucumbers, along with ornamental plants and flowers. The profit from the sales of these products is shared with all workers and reinvested into the farm.

Rights-based approaches to social work practice in mental health

Rights-based approaches to social work practice in mental health attend to everyone's right to mental health and to the human rights of people with mental disabilities (Dudley, Silove & Gale, 2012). These encompass the right to available, accessible, acceptable, and good quality mental health services, goods, facilities, and underlying determinants of mental health. Rights-based approaches to mental health value mental health, prevent mental disability, and promote the full range of human rights for people with mental disability. Rights-based social work practice in mental health should be community-based, non-discriminatory and universally accessible, participatory, transparent, and accountable to prevent rights violations in mental health care.

Rights-based approaches to social work affirm the human dignity and worth of people with mental disability (Gable & Gostin, 2004). Rights-based approaches require a paradigm shift that views people with mental disabilities as active, powerful, and full humans with unlimited potential, who are not required to prove their deservedness or to demonstrate their capability to exercise their rights (Burns, 2013; CSWE, 2011). Rights-based approaches do not view people with mental disabilities as deficient individuals but acknowledge the social, economic, and political conditions that interact with individual's physical, biological, mental, and psychological characteristics to produce a disability. Rights-based approaches draw from recovery, strengths-based, and person-in-environment perspectives on mental health, and support the right of people with mental disability to live, learn, work, and participate in their communities. People with mental disabilities are not passive consumers but active participants.

Rights-based approaches to social work practice do not focus on eliminating or reducing mental disability, but rather on the realization of human rights and full participation in society of people with mental disabilities. This is contrary to the medical model that implies a straightforward process of diagnosis, treatment, and cure.

Dignity means promoting self-determination, where a person with mental disability can exercise choice, define their own goals, and the pathway to achieving them. Social workers should maximize people with disabilities' autonomy and control of resources to achieve a self-determined life. Mental health is contingent upon confidence and personal efficacy; social workers must support the ability of people with disabilities to choose services and supports (CSWE, 2011). Rights-based approaches require practitioners to respect people with mental disabilities and treat them as equals, refraining from an "us versus them" hierarchical perspective. Social workers should respect the decisions of people with mental disabilities with compassion and empathy.

Social workers can promote the dignity of people with mental disabilities through psychiatric advance directives (Morrissey, 2010; Scheyett, Kim, Swanson & Swartz, 2007). Advance directives, or living wills, contain people's choices, decisions, and preferences about their care prior to needing to make any decisions; they are made during a time of mental capacity in anticipation of a later point of incapacitation. These tools could indicate treatment preferences of people with mental disabilities prior to a mental health crisis thus preserving some degree of their self-determination.

Rights-based approaches to social work practice must prioritize community integration; it is a human rights imperative for people with mental disabilities

(Hunt, 2005; WHO, 2001; Yamin & Rosenthal, 2005). Social workers should work for the fullest possible integration of people with mental disabilities in the community. This includes the right to live, to work, and to receive treatment and care through community-based services. Guided by the principle of services delivered in the "least restrictive environment", social work practice that supports community integration and community-based services contributes to the dignity, self-determination, equality, and participation of people with mental disabilities while diminishing discrimination. The more that people with mental disabilities live, work, and receive care in their communities, they less they will face stigma. Through community-based services, people with mental disabilities have demonstrated that they can experience recovery from mental disability, and enjoy independent living in the community. Community-based service models should be integrated into social work practice, mental health services, social service models, and general health systems.

Social workers have a prominent role to play in the provision and delivery of services for people with mental disabilities. Social workers can provide evidence-based practice guidelines, promote the recovery model of care, including alternatives to coercive programs, engage service-users and their families, and establish financing mechanisms for multi-sectoral intervention collaborations. Clinical interventions should focus on helping people with mental disabilities to explore, find, learn, practice, and adopt appropriate, healthy, and sustainable coping strategies in individual or group settings. Rights-based approaches include stress management, coping strategies, and exhibiting patience and empathy towards people with emotional challenges (Wronka, 2008). Services such as medication, psychotherapy, ambulatory services, hospitalization for acute care, residential facilities, rehabilitation, vocational training, independent living supports, supportive housing and employment, income support, inclusive and appropriate education, and respite care for caregivers should be available and accessible in the community in which the person with mental disability lives.

Rights-based approaches to social work practice focus on fighting against discrimination against people with disabilities, and prioritize eliminating disparities in mental health services and outcomes. Social workers must also prevent the denial of mental health care to anyone and exclusion from the underlying determinants of mental health. Rights-based social work practice with people with mental disability recognizes the deleterious effects of inequality, discrimination, stigma, and oppression that violate rights and contribute to poor mental health (Burns, 2013; CSWE, 2011; UN, 2008).

Rights-based approaches acknowledge that people with mental disabilities suffer more from the social conditions and cultural reactions that give rise to discrimination and stigma than by any physical or mental difference. That is, negative outcomes associated with people with mental disabilities such as isolation, poor health, poverty, and violence are more the result of an imbalance of power. This results in social conditions such as stigma, dependency, social exclusion, and barriers. Stigma contributes to underutilization and lack of access of mental health care and high rates of untreated and potentially unrecognized mental disability. The rights-based practice principle of nondiscrimination also means social workers must attend to mental health disparities.

Rights-based approaches, informed by the indivisibility of rights, should be holistic, integrative, individualized, and person-centered. Stigma and discrimination thrive where individual differences are overlooked; understanding a person's unique history and context can prevent practitioners from treating people as "cases" or "diagnoses". Holistic and integrative care involves multi-sectoral comprehensive community-based services across the life course. Rights-based mental health care should be community-based and integrated with maternal, sexual, reproductive, child health, HIV/AIDS, and chronic noncommunicable disease programs (WHO, 2013). This serves to normalize mental health within other settings and reduce stigma.

Social workers can combat discrimination by developing and delivering mental health care that promotes independence, autonomy, and self-determination, supports their social integration and inclusion, and prevents further disability or exclusion. Practitioners should work to elicit from people with disabilities their capabilities, resiliency, talents, coping skills, and strengths (CSWE, 2011; Saleeby, 1996). Rights-based approaches focus on integrating the whole person into society, rather than remedying some aspect of physical or mental limitation related to the disability.

People with mental disabilities have the right to mental health services that are acceptable to their cultural background; this refers to cultural competence, cultural sensitivity, and nondiscrimination (CSWE, 2011; Hunt, 2005). Rights-based approaches to mental health are respectful of cultural traditions; especially those of indigenous populations and ethnic, racial, and religious minorities. Cultural differences in the understanding and prevalence of mental disabilities and cultural variations on stigma and help-seeking behavior require rights-based approaches to tailor mental health services to culturally diverse populations. Social work assessment should attend to cultural and social diversity. Social workers should partner with and support community-based organizations catering to and specializing in diverse populations.

Rights-based social work practice must uphold the right of people with mental disabilities to participate in treatment, policy, and advocacy (Burns, 2013; CSWE, 2011). Participation is an expression of self-determination and a cornerstone of empowerment; participation resists paternalism and deficit-based models. This means promoting inclusive, user-driven services that incorporate the leadership of people with mental disabilities into policy and program design and delivery. Practitioners should engage with stakeholders such as peer-support groups, family members, and caregivers. Social workers should support the voices of the population that the system is supposed to serve in setting objectives, treatment planning, and evaluation.

Participation in processes and decisions that affect their mental health may sometimes be challenging for people with mental disabilities; this is not a justifiable reason to violate their rights but, rather, is why social workers must facilitate and support their participation and communication of their preferences and experiences. Participation can be challenging also when people with mental disabilities disagree with professionals in terms of their treatment decisions. Respecting the decision of a person with mental disability, even when the practitioner disagrees, is a key element of a rights-based approach. Social workers should strive to form partnerships with people with mental disabilities and avoid paternalistic models of practice. Participation of people with mental disabilities depends in part upon their capacity to engage and advocate for their needs with practitioners. Effective participation relies upon education. Social workers must make information available and educate people with mental disabilities about treatment and service options so they can make informed choices.

Organizations led by and comprised of people with mental disabilities must lead advocacy efforts; social workers should support these organizations and social movements, amplifying their voice to policymakers. This includes creating, strengthening, and working with representative organizations, such as self-help, consumer, family member, and caregiver groups to develop, implement, monitor, and reform mental health policies, programs, and practices that meet the needs and fulfill the rights of people with mental disabilities. User-led advocacy has a rich tradition in mental health. The disability rights and psychiatric survivors' movements have demonstrated how advocacy by people with mental disabilities can lead to legal and policy reforms, new services, and social transformations that have reduced discrimination (Goodley, 2005).

However, organizations that represent the interests of people with mental disabilities may not be well developed. Social workers should work to build the capacity of these organizations through technical assistance, networking, donor development, and fund-raising (CSWE, 2011). Civil society organizations of people with mental disabilities should be supported and expanded. Social workers should facilitate dialogue between these groups and human rights organizations, social work and professional organizations, education, health, employment, judiciary and other fields. Such organizations can consult to the Committee on the Rights of Persons with Disabilities, and lobby and assist states with mental health policies.

Participation in these organizations can foster social support for people with mental disabilities among their peers. Peer support involves the mutual sharing of experiential knowledge and skills and social learning. Social workers should enable people to access peer support for mutually reinforcing encouragement, sense of belonging, supportive relationships, valued roles, and community (Hodges, Hardiman & Segal, 2003).

The rights-based practice principle of transparency means that social workers must assess human rights violations against people with mental disabilities. Protecting people with mental disabilities from human rights violations includes preventing unnecessary institutionalization and mental health practices that have been abused in the past. Unfortunately, violations of the rights of people with mental disability still occur in mental health facilities, such as direct and unmodified electroconvulsive therapy without consent (Perlin, Cucolo & Ikehara, 2014; WHO, 2011). Transparency includes examining the risks of medicalizing psychosocial and mental disability and exporting psychiatric practices to the Global South, a form of medical colonization which may spread stigma and discrimination. Advocates have called for a public apology from states and mental health practitioners to the victims of psychiatric abuse for human rights violations committed in the name of treatment. Rights-based approaches recommend that practitioners respect advance directives, eliminate forced treatment, restraint, and seclusion practices (CSWE, 2011). Rights-based approaches can help clinicians respond to challenging behavior of people with mental disabilities in an ethical way, when competing rights are at stake (Bailey, Ridley & Greenhill, 2010).

Transparency in rights-based approaches to mental health relates to the accessibility of mental health goods, services, facilities, professionals, and medicines, including their affordability which is important given the prevalence of people with mental disabilities living in poverty and without access (Dudley, Silove & Gale, 2012). Transparency also refers to accessibility of information regarding rights, diagnosis, treatment, options, avenues for redress, and legal protections for people with mental disabilities. In the past, the mental health system has not been transparent for people with mental disabilities, due to an assumption of inability to comprehend. Transparency and access to information includes the right to mental health care of scientific, medical, and technological merit. This requires that practitioners be trained and educated on the best available scientific research, interventions, and procedures. Rights-based approaches include strengthening information systems and research capacity for mental health to ensure access to accurate mental health indicators and practice evidence.

People with mental disabilities have the right to know which interventions have benefited others, and to benefit from this knowledge. Ensuring that people with mental disabilities have access to transparent information regarding mental health policies, programs, and practices includes evidence-based practice, which requires users to be fully informed about any treatment or intervention they may undertake (CSWE, 2011; Hunt, 2006). The diversity of the population of people with mental disabilities precludes uniform applications of evidence-based practice. Effective evidence-based practice depends upon the service-user's input, being informed, and participating in their care. In rights-based approaches, practitioners should educate and share available information with service-users, empowering them to make informed decisions about their treatment. Knowledge about the efficacy and risks involved with treatment of people with mental disabilities facilitates their decision making, increases their autonomy, and realizes their right to informed consent. Dissemination of the latest evidence to practitioners should be a priority. Practitioners could develop a mental disability tribunal that reviews cases of psychiatric violations in order to protect the rights of people with mental disabilities (Perlin, Cucolo & Ikehara, 2014).

Transparency in mental assessments means that social workers should listen to individuals' understanding of their own condition, work as equal partners in their care, and offer choice in a range of treatments, interventions, and service providers.

Social workers should conduct rights-based assessments of mental health programs, focusing on the rights of people with mental disability to an adequate standard of living, health and mental health, liberty and security, freedom from degrading treatment, and to independent living in their community (WHO, 2013). Rights-based assessments should incorporate people with mental disabilities, include trainings on human rights for the service-users, family members, staff, and administrators, aim for the elimination of human rights violations in all facilities, improve the quality of care, lead to policy reforms, and build the capacity of service-users and practitioners. Social workers should strive to engage people with mental disabilities in constructing a global mental health research agenda to produce culturally validated best practices for realizing the right to mental health.

Rights-based approaches should prioritize prevention of mental disability. Early identification is especially important; children and adolescents with mental disability should be provided with evidence-based psychosocial and non-pharmacological interventions in community settings, which avoid institutionalization and medicalization. Prevention efforts should attend to the underlying determinants of mental health, including poverty, employment, education, health, family cohesion, and experiences of discrimination, human rights violations, and adverse life events including but not limited to sexual violence, child abuse, and neglect. Social workers should endeavor to reduce and limit exposure to environmental disasters, civil conflict, and armed group violence.

Prevention strategies include early childhood education; life skills and sex education; the promotion of safe, stable, and nurturing relationships between children and their families and care-givers; healthy living and working conditions, including evidence-based stress reduction and stress management programs; community protection networks for preventing child abuse, domestic violence, and community violence; and social protection. People with mental disabilities are susceptible to suicide; rights-based approaches to suicide prevention include reducing risk factors by restricting access to self-harm tools, promoting responsible media coverage of suicides, and supporting a robust mental health system.

The rights-based principle for practice of accountability in mental health legitimizes international scrutiny of national mental health policy and practices (Gable & Gostin, 2004). Individual approaches to the right to mental health are insufficient and must be complemented with advocacy in collaboration with people with mental disabilities (Burns, 2013).

Advocacy should engage stakeholders, including service-users, family members, human rights NGOs, faith-based organizations, mental health professionals, and social workers (WHO, 2010). Social workers should advocate for an adequate number of mental health goods, services, facilities, practitioners, and essential medicines. Rights-based policy reforms should include the provision of comprehensive, integrated mental health and social care services in community-based settings; strategies for promotion of non-discrimination, anti-stigma and prevention of mental disability; and coordination and strengthening of information systems, evidence, and research. Mental health policies should empower people with mental disabilities to make choices about their lives and participate in decisions about their care. Social workers should remove barriers to care, eliminate financial barriers, and promote mental health throughout society.

Social work practice should implicitly focus on changing the structural economic, social, and political factors that contribute to mental disabilities and ensure that people with mental disabilities enjoy the underlying determinants to mental health such as education, housing, water, food, and sanitation. Criminal justice reform should include reductions in incarceration rates, elimination of prolonged solitary confinement, and increasing access to mental health services in correctional facilities and for ex-prisoners (HRW, 2003).

Social workers should work to increase public investment in the rights of people with mental disabilities to maintain sufficient workforce, infrastructure, and program development. Practitioners, even in resource-poor environments, can implement positive reforms to advance the right to mental health. Examples of relatively low-cost programs include improving the training and education of all health, mental health, and social work professionals to emphasize respect, care, treatment, and the rights of people with mental disabilities; raising awareness through community education and public awareness campaigns against stigma and discrimination of people with mental disabilities; forming civil society organizations that are comprised of and represent mental health care users and their families; downsize psychiatric hospitals in favor of community-based care; the inclusion and participation of people with mental disabilities in the decisions and processes that affect them; and advocacy and lobbying for assistance and cooperation with donors and international organizations (Hunt, 2005).

Accountability for the right to mental health includes awareness and consciousness-raising and education campaigns in order to change the perceptions and attitudes that contribute to discrimination and stigma, publicize the availability of effective treatments and supports, and generate appreciation for the capacities and contributions of persons with disabilities (Burns, 2013). Social workers can develop and disseminate training materials on the rights of people with mental disability.

For further reading on rights-based approaches to mental health

Action on Disability and Development

NGO focused on nondiscrimination and development for people with disabilities in the Global South.
www.add.org.uk/

China Disabled Persons' Federation

National organization promoting full and equal participation of people with disabilities, founded by Deng Pufang, the 2003 recipient of the UN Prize in the field of Human Rights.
www.cdpf.org.cn/english/

Citizens Commission on Human Rights

A nonprofit mental health watchdog founded by Dr. Thomas Szasz working to raise awareness about the risks, viability, and alternatives to treatment.
www.cchr.org/

Disability Rights International

An NGO working on full participation and human rights for people with disabilities.
www.disabilityrightsintl.org/

Disabled People International

A cross–disability global disability people's organization.
www.dpi.org/

Mental Disability Advocacy Center

NGO promoting the right to community living for people with mental disabilities.
www.mdac.info/en

World Health Organization

WHO Department of Mental Health and Substance Abuse has a project on mental health
and human rights assisting states to protect the human rights of people with mental disorders. Website has country summaries for case studies.
www.who.int/mental_health/en/

References

Bailey, S., Ridley, J., Greenhill, B. (2010). Challenging behaviour: A human rights-based
approach. *Advances in mental health and intellectual disabilities, 4*(2), 20–26.
Burns, J. (2013). Mental health and inequity: A human rights approach to inequality, discrimination, and mental disability. *Health and Human Rights, 11*(2), 19–31.
Council on Social Work Education (CSWE). (2011). *Recovery to practice: Developing mental
health recovery in social work.* Alexandria, VA: Author. Retrieved from: www.cswe.org/File.
aspx?id=51135
Dudley, M., Silove, D., & Gale, F. (Eds.). (2012). *Mental health and human rights: Vision, praxis,
and courage.* Oxford: Oxford University Press.
Gable, L., & Gostin, L. (2009). Mental health as a human right. In A. Clapham, M. Robin-
son, C. Mahon, & S. Jerbi (Eds.), *Realizing the right to health* (pp. 249–261). Swiss Human
Rights Book (Vol. 3). Zurich: Ruffer & Rub.
Gambrill, E. (2012). *Propaganda in the helping professions.* Oxford: Oxford University Press.
Goodley, D. (2005). Empowerment, self-advocacy and resilience. *Journal of Intellectual Dis-
ability, 9*(4), 333–343.
Gostin, L., & Gable, L. (2004). The human rights of persons with mental disabilities: A global
perspective on the application of human rights principles to mental health. *Maryland Law
Review, 63*(20), 20–121.
Hodges, J., Hardiman, E., & Segal, S. (2003). Predictors of hope among members of mental
health self-help agencies. *Social Work in Mental Health, 2*(1), 1–16.
Human Rights Watch (HRW). (2003). *Ill-equipped: U.S. prisons and offenders with mental illness.*
New York: Author. Retrieved from: www.hrw.org/sites/default/files/reports/usa1003.pdf

Hunt, P. (2005). *Report of the Special Rapporteur on the right of everyone to the enjoyment of the highest attainable standard of physical and mental health. (Main focus: Mental disability and the right to health)*. E/CN.4/2005/51. Geneva: UN Office of the High Commissioner on Human Rights.

Hunt, P. (2006). *Report of the Special Rapporteur on the right of everyone to the enjoyment of the highest attainable standard of physical and mental health (Main focus: A human rights-based approach to health indicators)*. New York: UN Office of the High Commissioner for Human Rights. Retrieved from: http://daccess-dds-ny.un.org/doc/UNDOC/GEN/G06/114/69/PDF/G0611469.pdf?OpenElement

Katontoka, S. (2007). Users' networks for Africans with mental disorders. *Lancet, 370*(9591), 919–920.

Lecompt, J., & Mercier, C. (2007). The Montreal Declaration on Intellectual Disabilities of 2004: An important first step. *Journal of Policy and Practice in Intellectual Disabilities, 4*(1), 66–69.

Mental Disability Advocacy Center & Mental Health Users Network of Zambia (MDAC & MHUNZ). (2014). *Human rights and mental health in Zambia*. London: Author. Retrieved from: www.mdac.org/sites/mdac.info/files/zambia_layout_web4.pdf

Minkowitz, T., Galves, A., Brown, C., Kovary, M., & Remba, E. (2006). *Alternative Report on Forced Drugging, Forced Electroshock, and Mental Health Screen of Children in Violation of Article 7*. New York: Disability Working Group. Retrieved from: http://psychrights.org/Countries/UN/ICCPRfinaldisabilityreport.pdf

Morrissey, F. (2010). Advance directives in mental health care: Hearing the voice of the mentally ill. *Medico Legal Journal of Ireland, 21*(6), 1.

Morrissey, F. (2012). The United Nations Convention on the Rights of Persons with Disabilities: A new approach to decision-making in mental health law. *European Journal of Health Law, 19*(5), 423–440.

Oaks, D. (2007). MindFreedom International: Activism for human rights as the basis for a nonviolent revolution in the mental health system. In P. Stastny & P. Lehman (Eds.), *Alternatives beyond psychiatry* (pp. 328–336). Berlin: Peter Lehmann.

Oliver, M. (2009). *Understanding disability: From theory to practice* (2nd ed.). Basingstoke: Palgrave Macmillan.

Perlin, M., Cucolo, H., & Ikehara, Y. (2014). Online mental disability law education, a disability rights tribunal and the creation of an Asian disability law database: Their impact on research, training, and teaching of law, criminology, and criminal justice in Asia. *Asian Journal of Legal Studies, 1*(1), 15–31.

Rosenthal, E., & Rubenstein, L. (1993). International human rights advocacy under the 'Principles for the Protection of Persons with Mental Illness'. *International Journal of Law and Psychiatry, 16*(3–4), 257–300.

Saleeby, D. (1996). *The strengths perspective in social work practice*. New York: Longman.

Scheyett, A., Kim, M., Swanson, J., & Swartz, M. (2007). Psychiatric advance directives: A tool for consumer empowerment and recovery. *Psychiatric Rehabilitation Journal, 31*, 70–75.

Starnino, V. (2009). An integral approach to mental health recovery: Implications for social work. *Journal of Human Behavior in the Social Environment, 19*, 820–842.

Taylor, D. (2007). MindFreedom Ghana: Fighting for basic human conditions of psychiatric patients. In P. Stastny & P. Lehman (Eds.), *Alternatives beyond psychiatry* (pp. 336–342). Berlin: Peter Lehmann.

Torrey, E. (1997). Taking issue: Psychiatric survivors and nonsurvivors. *Psychiatric Services, 48*(2), 143.

Torrey, E. (2013). *American psychosis: How the federal government destroyed the mental illness treatment system*. Oxford: Oxford University Press.

United Nations (UN). (1991). *Principles for the Protection of Persons With Mental Illness and for the Improvement of Mental Health Care.* New York: Author. Retrieved from: www.un.org/documents/ga/res/46/a46r119.htm

United Nations (UN). (1993). *The Standard Rules on the Equalization of Opportunities for Persons with Disabilities.* New York: Author. Retrieved from: www.un.org/esa/socdev/enable/dissre00.htm

United Nations (UN). (1994). *General Comment No. 5: Persons With Disabilities.* New York: UN Committee on Economic, Social, and Cultural Rights. Retrieved from: http://tbinternet.ohchr.org/_layouts/treatybodyexternal/Download.aspx?symbolno=INT%2fCESCR%2fGEC%2f4760&Lang=en

United Nations (UN). (2000). *General Comment No. 14: The right to the highest attainable standard of health (Art. 12).* New York: UN Committee on Economic, Social and Cultural Rights. Retrieved from: http://tbinternet.ohchr.org/_layouts/treatybodyexternal/Download.aspx?symbolno=E%2fC.12%2f2000%2f4&Lang=en

United Nations (UN). (2002, April 8–12). *Madrid International Plan of Action on Ageing.* Second World Assembly on Ageing, Madrid, Spain. Retrieved from: http://undesadspd.org/Portals/0/ageing/documents/Fulltext-E.pdf

United Nations (UN). (2006). *Convention on the Rights of Persons with Disabilities.* New York: Author. Retrieved from: www.un.org/disabilities/convention/conventionfull.shtml

United Nations (UN). (2008). *Fact Sheet No. 31: The Right to Health.* Geneva: UN Office of the High Commissioner for Human Rights. Retrieved from: www.ohchr.org/Documents/Publications/Factsheet31.pdf

United Nations (UN). (2010). *General Recommendation No. 27: Older women and protection of their rights.* New York: UN Committee on the Elimination of Discrimination Against Women. Retrieved from: www2.ohchr.org/english/bodies/cedaw/docs/CEDAW-C-2010-47-GC1.pdf

World Health Organization (WHO). (2001). *World Health Report 2001: Mental health: New understanding, new hope.* Geneva: Author. Retrieved from: www.who.int/whr/2001/en/whr01_en.pdf?ua=1

World Health Organization (WHO). (2010). *Best practices: Mental health and development.* Geneva: Author. Retrieved from: www.who.int/mental_health/policy/development/mh_best_practices_development_2010_en.pdf

World Health Organization (WHO). (2011). *Mental health atlas.* Geneva: Author. Retrieved from: http://whqlibdoc.who.int/publications/2011/9799241564359_eng.pdf

World Health Organization. (2013). *Mental Health Action Plan 2013–2020.* Geneva: Author. Retrieved from: http://apps.who.int/iris/bitstream/10665/89966/1/9789241506021_eng.pdf?ua=1

World Network of Users and Survivors of Psychiatry (WNUSP). (2001). *Position paper on Principles for the Protection of Persons with Mental Illness.* Odense, Denmark: Author. Retrieved from: www.wnusp.net/index.php/position-paper-on-principles-for-the-protection-of-persons-with-mental-illness.html

Wronka, J. (2008). *Human rights and social justice: Social action and service for the helping and health professions.* Thousand Oaks, CA: Sage.

Yamin, E., & Rosenthal, E. (2005). Out of the shadows: Using human rights approaches to secure dignity and well-being for people with mental disabilities. *PLoS Medicine, 2*(4), 296–298.

8

PERILS AND PROSPECTS OF HUMAN RIGHTS-BASED APPROACHES TO SOCIAL WORK

This chapter concludes the book by reflecting on the perils and prospects of human rights for social work. The bulk of the chapter examines the limitations of rights-based approaches, both conceptually and practically. The final section looks forward to future directions for rights-based social work practice.

Perils and limits of human rights for social work

Human rights are a not a panacea for social work, the world, or for poverty, the suffering of children and older adults, ill health, and discrimination (Reichert, 2011). This book, while intended to encourage debate and examination of rights-based approaches to social work, is not meant to be naively optimistic about their potential. Human rights were acknowledged to be imperfect from the beginning, and even Eleanor Roosevelt was said to have called the Universal Declaration good but imperfect (Wronka, 2008).

As aspirational fields working to promote human well-being and social justice in an unjust world, human rights and social work face significant shortcomings. Both fields have experienced similar challenges along the way to achieving their mission and implementing their vision. Human rights are sometimes contested, as is social work, and have been subject to dismissive criticisms. The conceptual and practical limitations of human rights must be acknowledged with any consideration of rights-based approaches. There is insufficient space for a detailed discussion of these concerns; other scholars have tackled human rights' philosophical and theoretical limitations from a social work perspective (Ife, 2012; Reichert, 2011). Revisiting these debates is beyond the scope of this book; however, this analysis of rights-based approaches to social work practice would be remiss without some attention to the major critiques that have been raised.

Conceptual limits of rights-based approaches

Rights as rhetoric

It may be that rights-based approaches risk resulting in empty rhetoric; superficial changes to social work without deeper significance for practice. In the past, reform efforts in social work have generated initial excitement only to fail at solidifying into usable concepts or delivering practical tools. Human rights have been criticized as a distraction from the struggle for survival and the fulfillment of basic human needs and dismissed as "nonsense on stilts" (Jeremy Bentham cited in Wronka, 1998, p. 194). However it is because traditional approaches have failed to meet basic needs that rights-based approaches are called for. The elaboration of rights-based approaches to social work practice is meant to forestall a fad of human rights becoming buzzwords, by venturing into the realm of specific and practical applications.

Human rights and social work share a tension between engaging in lofty, idealistic rhetoric and making an authentic, meaningful difference in people's lives and their well-being. There is a utopianism to each field as practitioners seek to improve people's quality of life, and they can be prescriptive about how to accomplish their vision of a healthy or just world. This normative, prescriptive orientation can lead to practitioners feeling morally superior or justified, contributing to hierarchal relationships between those who know what is best and those who ought to be doing something different.

An undeniable limit of human rights is their propensity for convenient rhetoric covering self-righteousness. Human rights have been used to justify human rights violations. This is similar to how social work has been used to oppress vulnerable populations; this has been called the shadow side of social work (Sewpaul, 2014). The dynamic entails justification for intervention into another's affairs. Interventions may be well-intentioned and genuinely helpful, or they may be deceitfully self-serving and harmful. This has been called the "protection racket", and fits a pattern of Western exploitation; missionaries and colonists invaded in the name of dignity and oppressed under the cover of kindness. Social work is not immune from helping interventions that reinforce social stratification, reproduce oppression, and disempower people without sustainable improvements in their quality of life. Whenever human rights are proposed as justification for violating other's rights, issues of power must be considered (Ife, 2012). Rights-based approaches must include power analysis of structural privilege and disadvantage. These tendencies of both fields must be guarded against, and balanced with a commitment to local, indigenous, and bottom-up approaches.

Rights as imperfect obligations

Human rights are often conceptualized as entitlements, especially when rights are approached from a legal perspective which they commonly are. However, entitlements have limitations (Gable & Gostin, 2009). Entitlements imply legally binding obligations, requirements to respect, defend, and promote a right. Critics complain that human rights are frequently too vague to constitute an entitlement. For example, the right to mental health is difficult to define, implement, and to make justiciable. When rights lack operational and enforceable meanings, the entitlement approach is weakened. Further, entitlements are, in some states, a politically contested proposition. For example, in the U.S. entitlement programs are frequently targeted by fiscal conservatives for their expense.

Human rights have been dismissed as naive wish fulfillment on account of their unenforceability. Rights are often conceived as obligations upon states, who, even with all UN review mechanisms, are often operating on little more than a glorified honor system with little if any accountability to others on human rights issues. States are most often seen as the duty-bearers of rights, with obligations towards rights-holders. For this reason rights have been critiqued as unattainable and therefore not a worthwhile endeavor.

However, true as this may be, ultimately the people themselves are responsible for their institutions. States and formal institutions cannot exist without some degree of consent, from some people. This does not mean that the world is a populist paradise; far from it. Yet the will of the people is always a final recourse for human rights. This is why rights-based approaches almost always emphasize education towards a human rights culture, and why the principle of accountability must include community education as a key component.

Closer examination of so-called vague rights can reveal clear and justiciable elements, as the unpacking of the right to mental health in the last chapter revealed with the rights of people with mental disability to nondiscrimination, mental health services, and the underlying conditions which promote mental health. Also, concepts such as progressive realization help to diminish the conception of rights as purely entitlements; instead human rights are often a work in progress. Indeed, purely legal or policy definitions of rights as entitlements are insufficient; realizing rights requires practicing rights-based approaches.

Rights as static

Human rights have been criticized as legalistic abstractions divorced from the reality of ordinary people's daily lives. This criticism views human rights as static. To the contrary, human rights have a fluid dynamism that can touch the most personal and human experiences in everyday life (Wronka, 2008). The codification of human rights in documents belies their discursive nature and obscures the conversation, bargaining, negotiation, and consensus that human rights documents represent (Ife, 2012). Human rights are subject to debate and revision; they have been, and still can be, expanded to incorporate additional perspectives and rights.

Human rights were created by human beings; they are beset by human limitations (Wronka, 2008). Human rights are socially constructed; what it means to be human, who is considered human, and how to treat others is negotiated and renegotiated in daily life. Ultimately rights-based approaches are meant to humanize or re-humanize people who have been or who are at risk of dehumanization. Reconstructing rights into specific local and cultural contexts requires critical examination to prevent misapplication or mistranslation into practice (Reisch, 2014). Human rights can't be something that happens only in The Hague, or applied from afar in a one-size-fits all approach. For human rights to reach their full potential, they must be rooted in and relevant to people's immediate concerns, their homes, kitchens, and bedrooms; their work, offices, and schools; their humiliations and their pride (Roosevelt, 1958). Human rights must extend beyond practitioners' daily lives into their personal interactions with family, friends, associates, and strangers.

Rights as culture-bound

Human rights and social work both aspire to be universal in their relevance and application; however, both have been criticized for being culture-bound, products of social, political, and economic conditions (Wronka & Staub-Bernasconi, 2012). Both fields respond to core values that transcend place, boundary and border, gender, age, and class. Both fields also aspire to be applied locally and relevant to all people in all communities. Cultural relativism, which aims to equate all values and not privilege any one value over another, has also been criticized for privileging the value of relativism over all other values. The universalism of human rights is not meant to be "one size fits all", but rather universally inclusive and not based on any category that has been used to determine status or rights in the past. The philosophical debate may be overwrought; human rights are meant to be universal, relative to all cultures. Cultural relativism is meant to apply universally to all cultures.

Human rights are germane to all cultures. Regional human rights agreements from every corner of the globe have endorsed the universality of human rights, and many diverse people locate the basis for the ethical claims of human rights within their own indigenous cultural and religious traditions (Wronka & Staub-Bernasconi, 2012). There is widespread agreement on the principles and goals of human rights; the UDHR is consistent with religious, ethical, and value traditions of multiple cultures around the world (Reichert, 2011; Wronka, 2008). This is true in terms of the five principles of rights-based practice approaches. However, questions emerge during the application process: how to implement and enforce rights, under what conditions they are abridged and compromised, when do the rights of the community outweigh the rights of individuals?

Human need has been proposed as the universal aspect of human rights and social work, superseding cultural limitations (Wronka & Staub-Bernasconi, 2012). While need is universal, the means and modes of need fulfillment are cultural. This book will not pretend to resolve these issues, but rather has explored interpretations and applications of human rights to specific social work contexts. As with social work ethics, the solution lies in careful interpretation of universal values within a local cultural context; this is a central task of cultural competence. Cultural practices that violate human rights should be questioned; however the human right to one's own culture cautions would-be champions to proceed with cultural humility.

Human rights judgments, despite the valuable tactic of naming and shaming, are ripe for hypocrisy; no culture or society is free from human rights violations. Human rights should not be the basis for divisiveness, but rather a method for uniting diverse traditions in the pursuit of human dignity (Ife, 2012). Human rights are sufficiently inclusive for everyone; diversity and universality are not contradictory.

Rights-based approaches should attend to dynamics of inclusion and exclusion; unpacking whose voices are determining which rights are prioritized and how. To ensure that no one is excluded from rights-based approaches, practitioners should seek viewpoints that counter perceived mainstream perspectives and investigate negative space by asking who is not being included. This relates to the principles of participation and transparency. Interestingly, rights-based approaches have been extended through time; backwards via apologies, memorials, and transitional justice and forwards via intergenerational conflict, children's right to the future, and environmental sustainability (Ife, 2012).

Rights as Western

Universalism and globalism become problematically top-down when the West announces what the rest of the world must adopt. Are human rights just an extension of an individualistic approach that is anathema to non-Western societies and communities? Both human rights and social work are historically related to the Enlightenment project of modernity. Human rights have been traced to historical shifts in Europe wherein individual liberty became the paramount shape of political, legal, and economic systems. The concern is that Western approaches ought not to apply to other regions, and that individual approaches are inappropriate in many places. Critics also warn that human rights constitute moral imperialism of the West to the rest (Ignatieff, 2001). Social work also has a history of professional imperialism (Midgley, 1981). Human rights and social work can unintentionally recreate the harmful relationships of imperialism or colonialism. However, human rights have been employed by many to support families, communities, and social groups in non-Western societies. Despite their origin, human rights have emerged as a tool for oppressed minorities to fight for power against repressive regimes and exploitative corporations.

Rights as conflicting priorities

Human rights have been criticized for presenting conflicting priorities which the rights paradigm cannot resolve. This critique suggests that the principle of indivisibility breaks down during implementation when conflicting rights are pitted against each other (Wronka & Staub-Bernasconi, 2012). This is often referred to as the indivisibility versus hierarchy of rights debate. The contested nature of choosing which rights to prioritize or to implement over others is partially the reason for the civil-political and economic-social-cultural split between generations of rights. Rights-based approaches must balance conflicting rights; social work practice similarly requires the balancing of ethics. In practice, conflicting rights require analysis of power relations, in order to avoid the privileging of the rights of the powerful and marginalizing those whose rights have been violated.

Another criticism is that some rights are more accessible, defensible, justiciable, or affordable than others. Typically civil and political rights have been identified as such, contributing to their prominence over economic, social, and cultural rights. This book, approaching human rights from a social work perspective, has employed an integrative model for practice in each domain. All human rights are comprehensively examined from the perspective of a specific practice area such as health. For example, the right to health is predicated upon the right to be free from torture as much as the right to accessible medical care, and the right to water, as denial of water is a form of torture, and insufficient water has adverse health consequences.

This novel integrative approach avoids the historical and political baggage that divides human rights and blunts the development of rights-based practice. This integrative model is based on the indivisibility and non-hierarchy of human rights; civil rights are interdependent with economic rights. All three generations of rights apply to social work; all three should be incorporated into practice. Indivisibility mirrors intersectionality; because the problems are indivisible, the solutions must be indivisible. Rights-based approaches that integrate the indivisibility of rights are appropriate responses to the intersectionality of oppression. It is the intersection of gender and racial discrimination that mutually reinforce the oppression of women of color; therefore rights-based approaches must address equally the human rights of women and racial minorities.

Rights as social justice

Human rights and social justice are frequently used together, especially by social workers. Despite having significant overlap, these terms are sometimes confused or used in synonymy. Distinctions have been made between their respective focuses and tools (Marks, 2013; Wronka, 2008). Social justice has been characterized by a focus on the negative influence of structural conditions and global inequality on marginalized communities through the use of social mobilization and community development to balance economic globalization. Human rights have been characterized as focusing on developing and enforcing an accountability framework through legalistic means, referring to explicit human rights norms rather than ideological concepts of justice. Human rights, when concerned with individual claims against authority, can be seen as narrower social justice claims for redressing broad injustice. These distinctions are arbitrary, as human rights has been applied to broad global concerns, and social justice has been related to individuals and clinical practice. Social workers have used both legal advocacy for social justice and community education for human rights.

Social justice has also been articulated as a greater priority than human rights for social workers (Reisch, 2014). This has led to concern that more fully integrating human rights into social work could hamper the pursuit of social justice. The broad acceptance of the social justice concept among U.S. social workers may contribute to less general acceptance of human rights (NASW, 2008; Reichert, 2011). This is reinforced by historical and cultural bias toward civil and political rights over economic, social, and cultural rights.

However, social justice has been critiqued as ill-defined and misused without contemporary relevance (Reichert, 2011). The lack of consensus on its meaning and implementation dilutes the concept's value. In contrast, human rights are specifically defined, enumerated, articulated, and publicized in numerous human rights documents, treaties, and conventions, and then interpreted through general comments. Social justice may be best viewed as a vision or goal, while human rights, especially considering rights-based approaches, can be thought of as the means to achieve social justice. In this sense, social justice is the condition when all human rights are realized and protected (Midgley, 2007).

Viewing rights through a justice lens also raises the tension between seeking justice and caring for people's needs. A rights-based perspective offers a critique of humanitarian aid when presented as apolitical and sanitized. The need for care is frequently the result of human rights violations; a rights-based approach to aid maintains that future violations should be prevented by making perpetrators accountable. However, some NGOs such as the Red Cross utilize a strict neutral stance to gain access to the most vulnerable people.

Social work has long struggled with the tension between cause and function (Lee, 1937) and has been criticized for overemphasizing providing care over seeking justice (Specht & Courtney, 1994). Practice is care-oriented when it is remedial and focused on assisting individuals to adapt to their environments; preventative, community organization, or policy practice focused on changing the social environment to better accommodate people is justice-oriented.

Practical limits of rights-based approaches

Human rights are beset by gaps between idealized aspirations and disappointing realities (Fredvang & Biggs, 2012). Widespread consensus on the goals of human rights has not yielded agreement on the process to achieve the goals. This section discusses related practical limitations of implementing rights-based approaches. These flaws dos not render rights invalid or unrealizable.

Limits of practice

It has been argued that specifying rights-based approaches diminishes the complex nature of human rights, and that their power is derived in part from sorting through this complexity (Ife, 2012). Prescriptive models for practitioners oversimplify human rights. Approaches that reduce principles into practice risk becoming one-size-fits-all approaches that are contrary to the spirit of human rights. Critics say that rights-based approaches define human rights for others, which violates participatory processes of dialogue and consensus.

However, this ignores the great deal of dialogue that has occurred on how to implement human rights principles. There is great value in examining ways that social workers can incorporate human rights into their practice; remaining ignorant of other fields' progress in applying rights-based approaches limits the sustainability of the profession. Simply telling social workers to advance human rights will not effect change; concrete guidance for incorporating human rights into practice is critical.

Limits of states as duty-bearers

Critics of international human rights mechanisms complain that it is unrealistic to place too much responsibility upon states beset with myriad economic, political, and social problems (Tang & Lee, 2006). Even when states have agreed to international standards, they may fail to establish domestic policies, institutions, or programs to fulfill their commitment (Fredvang & Biggs, 2012). The principle of progressive realization, contained in many international human rights standards, acknowledges that state resources are not uniform and permits the gradual realization of rights over time.

Human rights have been criticized for their lack of enforcement, diminishing their potential (Reichert, 2011). If states are the primary duty-bearers, then the question becomes who has the authority and the power to hold a state government accountable for its human rights obligations. States mostly police themselves by their own consent. State implementation gaps are frequently analyzed in shadow reports through comparisons of international commitments, their statements of reservation at the time of signing agreements, and their social policies.

Despite the primacy of states as duty-bearers, responsibility and obligations should be understood to apply to everyone, including economic actors such as multinational corporations, civil society, and an active, educated, informed, and developed people and their institutions (Wronka & Staub-Bernasconi, 2012). Ideally, everyone should publicize human rights issues and pressure unresponsive states. Human rights are not guarantees, but tools, which all people, including social workers, can use.

Human rights can be used as measuring sticks, indicators of misery or progress. Unfortunately much of the human rights discourse is limited by a violation-accountability dynamic, consisting of moralizing through the naming and shaming of perpetrators, hoping that they will stop or be stopped. While this is important work, rights-based approaches require more; the conceptualization and implementation of human rights solutions.

Limits of implementing rights

Human rights have been called imperfect obligations for their over-reliance on unaccountable states, challenges in enforcing rights, and difficulty realizing rights-based approaches (Sengupta, Negi & Basu, 2006). Adopting rights-based approaches may result in unintended consequences for agencies, organizations, programs and the people they serve (Kindornay, Ron & Carpenter, 2012).

There is evidence that some social workers identify with the rhetoric of the strengths-based approach while actually practicing from a deficit-based approach (CSWE, 2011). To be sure, incorporating rights-based approaches into social work practice will require significant organizational transition including investment from administrators and practitioners.

Rights-based principles for practice, especially participation, transparency, and accountability, may place substantial excess burden upon practitioners and organizations. Participation requires the time and energy of local people that may exceed their capacity; transparency might mean that organizations assume additional research and monitoring tasks requiring significant additional documentation; accountability may be especially challenging for service-oriented organizations. Increased advocacy or education efforts may result in less service delivery, leading to loss of popular support and even participation from local constituencies. Management and staff may resist or make only superficial changes. This would risk turning rights-based approaches into empty promises, easily dismissed for a new approach.

To maximize the impact of rights-based approaches, vague definitions of various human rights should be reconciled and used with precision. Buy-in from key stakeholders is essential, including institutions such as social work professional organizations and education departments, and subgroups within these such as administrators, faculty, and field instructors.

Prospects for human rights-based approaches in social work

Rights-based approaches have much value to offer social work, including adding public focus to an increasingly private oriented profession preoccupied with micro therapies, behavioral modification, and symptom management (Specht & Courtney, 1994; Staub-Bernasconi, 2007). A human rights perspective connects individual ills to public issues and debates. Some have pointed to human rights as a way to rescue the social justice imperative of the social work profession.

Human rights are dynamic and evolving. So, too, are rights-based approaches; these are constantly being revised as new understandings and approaches are discovered (Gatenio Gabel, 2015). In addition to core fields of social work practice, rights-based approaches are relevant to various modes of practice. Previous chapters have endeavored to emphasize the relevance of rights-based approaches to specific fields or populations over a range of micro and macro levels of interventions. However, this section considers rights-based approaches for specific modes of practice.

Macro practice

Rights-based approaches have been identified as particularly salient for community practice (Libal & Harding, 2015), and rights-based approaches to administration and management (Wronka, 2008) and social policy (Gatenio Gabel, Harding, Libal,

Mapp & Androff, 2013) have been presented. Market-based approaches are becoming very popular (Anderson, 2014). The UN is increasingly engaging with for-profit organizations on human rights, through the Global Compact program. In social work, macro practice has a proud history dating to engagement with and support for the Universal Declaration. However, macro practice has shrunk in proportion to micro practice within the profession (Rothman & Mizrahi, 2014). Already under threat, macro practice is not sufficiently robust to integrate rights-based approaches within the entire profession of social work; human rights must be made relevant to all social workers.

Research

Research has a fundamental role in rights-based approaches. A rights-based approach to social work research would promote human dignity; be nondiscriminatory and transparent; include the participation of the people being studied; and contribute to accountability. Rights-based research pertains to research ethics, impact assessments, program evaluation, and participatory methods. Access to scientific research is itself a human right (Chapman, 2013). Ethical research is based on human rights (Wronka, 2008). The rights of research participants typically include informed consent and protection from harm. These are related to the practice principle of human dignity; informed consent is an expression of self-determination in research studies. The protection of research participants from harm also relates to nondiscrimination. Rights-based approaches to program evaluation for social workers means attending to the duty of care, trust-building, proactive collaboration, lifting the voices of participants, storytelling, attending to themes of oppression and marginalization, attending to "endings" of relationships, and preventing vicarious trauma (McNamara, 2013). Social work research should also conduct human rights impact studies that could build upon environmental impact studies to assess how new policies or programs will affect human rights (Wronka, 2008). Social work research should also evaluate rights-based approaches in practice and programs. These measures incorporate the principle of transparency through contributing clarity about impact, outcomes, and effectiveness. Participatory action research methods are especially relevant to rights-based research and embody the principle of participation.

Additional future directions

This book has only sketched rights-based approaches for a few practice areas; however, the principles of rights-based practice can be applied to rights-based approaches in diverse settings with myriad populations. Rights-based approaches can be used in both local and global contexts. Some areas are obvious for rights-based social work, such as with victims of torture or human trafficking (Androff, 2011). Other areas may seem more mundane but are no less relevant to human rights. Social workers can address homelessness from a human rights perspective by focusing on housing rights. For example, in the "housing first" model social workers focus on the right of people who are homeless to adequate housing instead of utilizing temporary or transitional housing and focusing on behavioral changes.

Social workers can use human rights-based approaches in relation to crime, conflict resolution, and violence prevention. Social workers have long been involved in the criminal justice system. Human rights touch every aspect of criminal justice; victims of violence have suffered violations of civil and political rights, and frequently their rights to health and mental health, among others. Incarcerated people have rights which are frequently overlooked. Social work has long been concerned with promoting peace and ending violence. Rights-based approaches are appropriate for social workers addressing large and small scale violence, from genocide to intimate partner violence. Rights-based approaches to crime and violence include narrative therapy (Androff, 2012c; Androff & McPherson, 2014; McPherson, 2012), restorative justice (Androff, 2012a; 2010b), and transitional justice mechanisms for transparency and accountability such as Truth and Reconciliation Commissions (Androff, 2010a; 2012b). The tools can also be applied to protecting the rights of human rights defenders, including social workers who are advancing human rights.

Global migration is an area ripe for rights-based social work practice with immigrants, migrant workers, and refugees. Immigrants face violations of the right to life (Androff & Tavassoli, 2012), fair working conditions (Ayón, Moya-Salas, Gurrola & Androff, 2012), and access to education, health and social services (Becerra, Androff, Ayón, Castillo, 2012). Immigration policies and border security measures can violate human rights (Androff, 2014); children's rights are frequently threatened by anti-immigrant policies (Androff et al., 2011).

Social workers should utilize rights-based approaches in practice with indigenous people around the world. Rights-based approaches to social work practice are also relevant to new forms of practice such as green social work that promotes environmental justice in the wake of climate change, disasters both natural and human caused, and environmental degradation (Androff, Fike & Rorke, in press). Vulnerable populations such as children and people living in poverty are particularly susceptible to health consequences of violations of the rights to food, water, sanitation, and underlying environmental conditions.

Social work's contribution to human rights

This book has explored how human rights can have a greater impact upon social work through rights-based approaches to social work practice. The converse is also true: social work has a lot to offer the field of human rights. Social work's messy and inspired practical application yields important implications for human rights. Social workers' focus on delivering social care and their role as instruments implementing social policy is unlikely to recede; therefore, their potential for advancing human rights is great. Social work expertise in building strong individuals families and communities can protect and fulfill human rights; social workers are front-line economic, social, and cultural rights workers. Social workers respect self-determination, human diversity, and indivisibility. Many practitioners incorporate these across interventions as basic aspects of their work. Social work values and interventions can contribute a community-based, empowering, and participatory perspective to the human rights field.

Social work has an enormous opportunity to embrace and impact human rights. The incorporation of human rights in social work curricula, research, and practice, will position the profession to contribute to the realization of human rights and to the human rights movement.

References

Anderson, S. (2014). *New strategies for social innovation: Market-based approaches for assisting the poor*. New York: Columbia University Press.

Androff, D. (2010a). Truth and reconciliation commissions (TRCs): An international human rights intervention and its connection to social work. *British Journal of Social Work, 40*(6), 1960–1977.

Androff, D. (2010b). 'To not hate': Reconciliation among victims of violence and participants of the Greensboro Truth and Reconciliation Commission. *Contemporary Justice Review, 13*(3), 269–285.

Androff, D. (2011). The problem of contemporary slavery: An international human rights challenge for social work. *International Social Work, 54*(2), 209–222.

Androff, D. (2012a). Adaptations of truth and reconciliation commissions in the North American context: Local examples of a global restorative justice intervention. *Advances in Social Work: Special Issue on Global Problems and Local Solutions, 13*(2), 408–419.

Androff, D. (2012b). Can civil society reclaim the truth? Results from a community-based truth and reconciliation commission. *International Journal of Transitional Justice, 6*(2), 296–317.

Androff, D. (2012c). Narrative healing among victims of violence: The impact of the Greensboro Truth and Reconciliation Commission. *Families in Society, 93*(1), 10–16.

Androff, D. (2014). Human rights and the war on immigration. In R. Furman & A. Akerman (Eds.), *Criminalization of immigration: Contexts and consequences*. Durham, NC: Carolina Academic Press.

Androff, D., Ayón, C., Becerra, D., Gurrola, M., Salas, L., Krysik, J., Gerdes, K., & Segal, E. (2011). US immigration policy and immigrant children's well-being: The impact of policy shifts. *Journal of Sociology and Social Welfare, 38*(1), 77–98.

Androff, D., Fike, C., & Rorke, J. (in press). Greening social work education: Teaching environmental rights and sustainability in community practice. *Journal of Social Work Education*.

Androff, D., & McPherson, J. (2014). Can human rights-based social work practice bridge the micro/macro divide? In K. Libal, M. Berthold, R. Thomas, & L. Healy (Eds.), *Advancing human rights in social work education* (pp. 23–40). Alexandria, VA: CSWE Press.

Androff, D., & Tavassoli, K. (2012). Deaths in the desert: The human rights crisis on the US-Mexico border. *Social Work, 57*(2), 165–173.

Ayón, C., Moya-Salas, L., Gurrola, M., & Androff, D. (2012). Intended and unintended consequences of employer sanction laws on Latino families. *Qualitative Social Work, 11*(6), 587–603.

Becerra, D., Androff, D., Ayón, C., & Castillo, J. (2012). Fear vs. facts: Examining the economic impact of undocumented immigrants in the U.S. *Journal of Sociology and Social Welfare, 39*(4), 111–134.

Chapman, A. (2013). Human rights: A human right to science. *Science, 341*(6148), 841–842.

Council on Social Work Education (CSWE). (2011). *Recovery to practice: Developing mental health recovery in social work.* Alexandria, VA: Author. Retrieved from: www.cswe.org/File. aspx?id=51135

Fredvang, M., & Biggs, S. (2012). *The rights of older persons: Protection and gaps under human rights law.* Social Policy Working Paper no. 16. Centre for Public Policy & Brotherhood of St. Laurence. Melbourne: University of Melbourne. Retrieved from: http://social. un.org/ageing-working-group/documents/fourth/Rightsofolderpersons.pdf

Gable, L., & Gostin, L. (2009). Mental health as a human right. In A. Clapham, M. Robinson, C. Mahon, & S. Jerbi (Eds.), *Realizing the right to health* (pp. 249–261). Swiss Human Rights Book (Vol. 3). Zurich: Ruffer & Rub.

Gatenio Gabel, S. (2015). Foreword, in K. Libal & S. Harding, Rights-based approaches to community practice (pp. v–xv). In S. Gatenio Gabel (Ed.), *Springer briefs in rights-based approaches to social work.* New York: Springer.

Gatenio Gabel, S., Harding S., Libal, K., Mapp, S., & Androff, D. (2013, June 19). *A rights-based approach to social policies.* Symposia on Human Rights and Social Policy. Global Health and Well-Being: The Social Work Response. New York University, New York.

Ife, J. (2012). *Human rights and social work: Towards rights-based practice* (3rd ed.). Cambridge: Cambridge University Press.

Ignatieff, M. (2001). *Human rights as politics and idolatry.* Princeton, NJ: Princeton University Press.

Kindornay, S., Ron, J., & Carpenter, C. (2012). Rights-based approaches to development: Implications for NGOs. *Human Rights Quarterly, 34*(2), 472–506.

Lee, P. (1937). *Social work as cause and function.* New York: Columbia University Press.

Libal, K., & Harding, S. (2015). Human rights-based community practice in the United States. In S. Gatenio Gabel (Ed.), *Springer briefs in rights-based approaches to social work series.* New York: Springer.

Marks, S. (2013). Poverty. In D. Moeckli, S. Shah, & S. Sivakumaran (Eds.), *International human rights law* (2nd ed., pp. 602–621). Oxford: Oxford University Press.

McNamara, P. (2013). Giving voice to children and young people in research: Applying rights-based frameworks to meet ethical challenges. *Developing Practice, 37,* 55–66.

McPherson, J. (2012). Does narrative exposure therapy reduce PTSD in survivors of mass violence? *Research in Social Work Practice, 22,* 29–42.

Midgley, J. (1981). *Professional imperialism: Social work in the third world.* London: Heinemann.

Midgley, J. (2007). Development, social development, and human rights. In E. Reichert (Ed.), *Challenges in human rights* (pp. 97–121). New York: Columbia University Press.

National Association of Social Workers (NASW). (2008). *Code of Ethics.* Washington, DC: Author. Retrieved from: www.socialworkers.org/pubs/code/code.asp

Reichert, E. (2011). *Social work and human rights: A foundation for policy* (2nd ed.). New York: Columbia University Press.

Reisch, M. (2014). The boundaries of social justice: Addressing the conflict between human rights and multiculturalism in social work education. In K. Libal, M. Berthold, R. Thomas, & L. Healy (Eds.), *Advancing human rights in social work education.* Alexandria, VA: CSWE Press.

Roosevelt, E. (1958, March 27). *In your hands: A guide for community action for the tenth anniversary of the Universal Declaration of Human Rights.* Retrieved from: www.un.org/en/ globalissues/briefingpapers/humanrights/quotes.shtml

Rothman, J., & Mizrahi, T. (2014). Balancing micro and macro practice: A challenge for social work. *Social Work, 59*(1), 91–93.

Sengupta, A., Negi, A., & Basu, M. (Eds.). (2006). *Reflections on the right to development.* Thousand Oaks, CA: Sage.

Sewpaul,V. (2014, July 11). *Politics with soul: Social work and the legacy of Nelson Mandela.* Eileen Younghusband Lecture at the 3rd Joint World Conference of Social Work and Social Development, Melbourne, Australia.

Specht, H., & Courtney, M. (1994). *Unfaithful angles: How social work has abandoned its mission.* New York: Free Press.

Tang, K., & Lee, J. (2006). Global social justice for older people: The case for an international convention on the rights of older people. *British Journal of Social Work, 36*(7), 1135–1150.

Wronka, J. (1998). *Human rights and social policy in the 21st century: A history of the idea of human rights and comparison of the United Nations Universal Declaration of Human Rights with United States federal and state constitutions* (Rev. ed.). Lanham, MD: University Press of America.

Wronka, J. (2008). *Human rights and social justice: Social action and service for the helping and health professions.* Thousand Oaks, CA: Sage.

Wronka, J., & Staub-Bernasconi, S. (2012). Human rights. In K. Lyons, T. Hokenstad, M. Pawar, N. Huegler, & N. Hall (Eds.), *The SAGE handbook of international social work* (pp. 70–84). Thousand Oaks, CA: Sage.

INDEX

National Association of Social Workers (NASW) 63; *Code of Ethics* 3, 13, 35, 37, 39, 41
nondiscrimination 37–40; children 74, 81, 83; health 109, 111, 117; mental health 128, 135; older adults 94–6, 101–2; poverty 64–5
Nussbaum, Martha 51

Ohio State University 9
older adults 88–106; accountability 98, 102; case study of rights-based approaches 99–100; conceptions of aging 89; consequences associated with aging 89–90; further reading 104; global demographics 88–91; human rights 92–8; rights-based approaches to social work practice 100–3; traditional approaches 91–2; *see also* Convention on the Elimination of All Forms of Discrimination against Women: older adults; Convention on the Rights of Older Persons; HelpAge International; International Covenant on Civil and Political Rights: older adults; Madrid International Plan of Action on Ageing; Universal Declaration of Human Rights: older adults
Optional Protocols to the Convention on the Rights of the Child 77
Organization of American States 63
Oxfam International 65

Pan-American Health Organization 127
participation 11, 27, 34, 38, 41–2; children 75, 81, 83–4; health 115–6, 118; mental health 130–5; older adults 99, 102; poverty 66
People's Health Movement – India 116
perils and prospects of human rights-based approaches to social work 143–56; conceptual limits 144–9; future directions 152–3; limits of implementing rights 150–1; limits of practice 149–50; limits of states as duty-bearers 150; macro practice 151–2; perils and limits of human rights for social work 143–51; practical limits of rights-based approaches 149–51; prospects for human rights-based approaches in social work 151–2; research 152; rights as conflicting priorities 147–8; rights as culture-bound 146–7; rights as imperfect

obligations 144–5; rights as rhetoric 144; rights as social justice 148–9; rights as static 145–6; rights as Western 147; social work's contribution to human rights 153–4
personal-professional model 30–1
Physicians for Human Rights 120
PLAN International 79
policy practice 10, 31–2, 43, 84, 102, 117, 149
Poor People's Economic Human Rights Campaign (PPEHRC) 63–5
poverty 50–70; absolute measure 51, 52; accountability 65, 66–7; additional mechanisms relating to 62–3; case study 63–5; conceptions 50–1; declining global trend 53; extent 52–4; further reading 67; global estimates 52; human right to be free from 56–9; inequality 53; outliers 53; regional estimates 52–3; rights-based approaches to social work practice 65–7; right to development 59–62; traditional approaches 54–6; what social workers need to know 56–8; *see also* International Covenant on Economic, Social and Cultural Rights; Millennium Development Goals; Poor People's Economic Human Rights Campaign; Universal Declaration of Human Rights: poverty
PPEHRC *see* Poor People's Economic Human Rights Campaign
principles of rights-based social work practice 34–45; accountability 43–5; human dignity 34–7; nondiscrimination 37–40; participation 41–2; transparency 42–3
Protocol of San Salvador 63, 96, 116
Protocol to the African Charter on the Rights of Women in Africa 96

Reichert, Elisabeth 6
REPLACE Campaign 86
Research and Training Centre for Community Development (RTCCD) 115
Reynolds, Bertha Capen 11–2
Richmond, Mary: *Social Diagnosis* 107
Right of Everyone to the Enjoyment of the Highest Attainable Standard of Physical and Mental Health 113, 129
rights-based approaches to social work practice 27–33; child welfare 83; existing models 27–8; health 116; holistic micro